Where Dreams Come Alive

The Alchemy of the African Healer

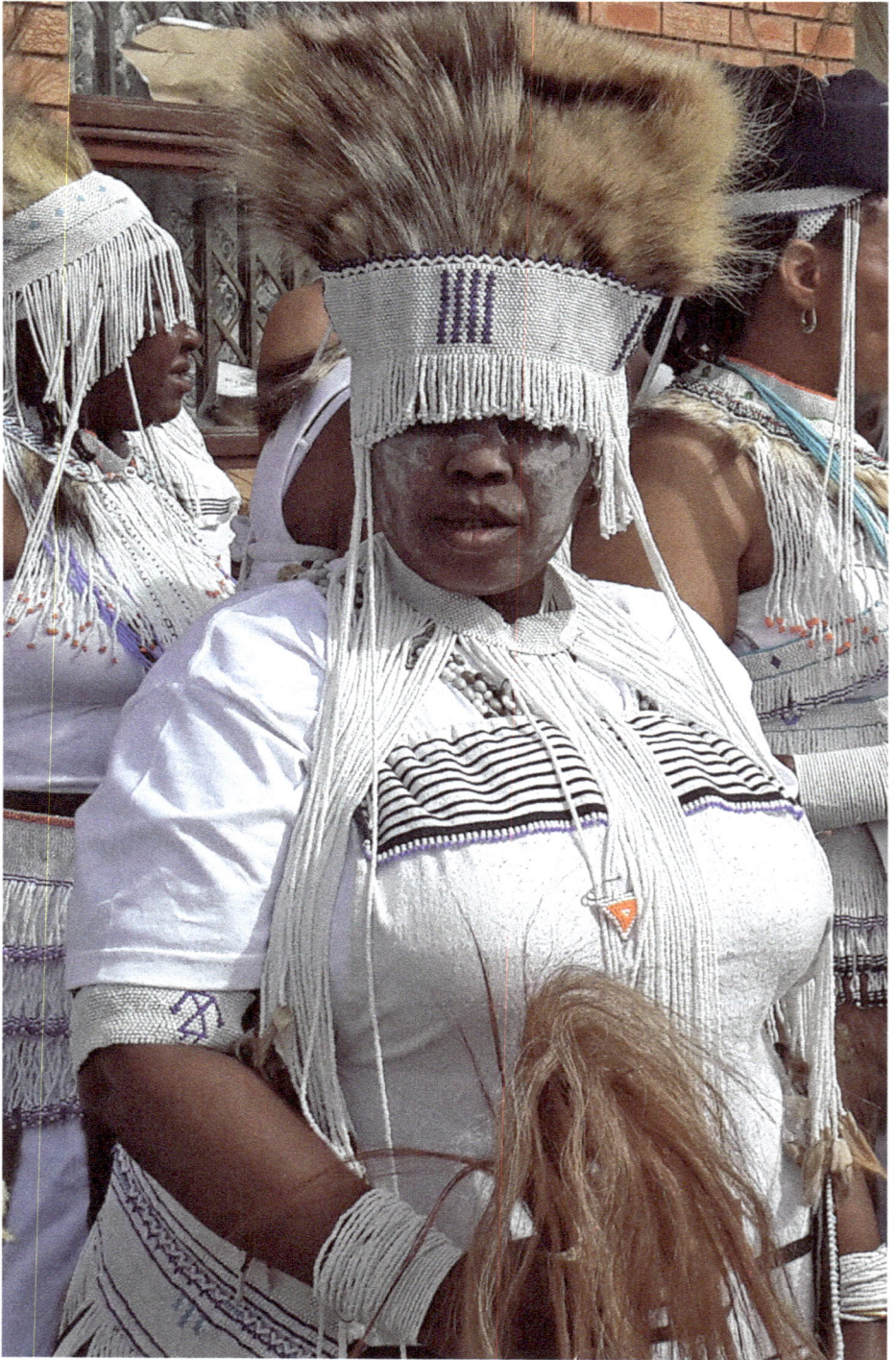

An Initiate displays the intricate bead work of her regalia
during the whitening stage of the initiation

Where Dreams Come Alive

The Alchemy of the African Healer

LYNNE RADOMSKY

CHIRON PUBLICATIONS • ASHEVILLE, NORTH CAROLINA

www.ChironPublications.com

Interior and cover design by Danijela Mijailovic
Printed primarily in the United States of America.

COVER IMAGE © Author: A *sangoma* dances during an initiation ritual displaying the regalia of a senior healer including the animal skin, bead work and gallbladders on her head.

Interior images taken by author, unless otherwise noted.

Permission from Princeton University Press, provided by Copyright Clearance Center to reproduce images from:
C.G. Jung (1944/1968). *Psychology and alchemy*, *CW*, vol. 12. Princeton University Press

Interior figures in MS from Jung, CW, vol. 12: Figure 17: Part 111, Chapter 1, fig. 114; Figure 38: Part 11, Chapter 5, fig. 30; Figure 42: Part 111, Chapter 5, fig. 230

IMAGES FROM MUTUS LIBER: Altus & Tollé. (1702) *Mutus Liber*: [Genevae? [s.n.] 1702][Pdf] Retrieved from The Library of Congress http://www.loc.gov/item/100184321. Public Domain Mark 1.0@1raci : Accessed on 11 November 2018

Interior figures in MS from MUTUS LIBER: Figure 25, Figure 30, Figure 39, Figure 40, Figure 48

ISBN 978-1-63051-708-3 paperback
ISBN 978-1-63051-709-0 hardcover
ISBN 978-1-63051-711-3 limited edition paperback

Library of Congress Cataloging-in-Publication Data

Names: Radomsky, Lynne, author.
Title: Where dreams come alive : the alchemy of the African healer / Lynne Radomsky.
Description: Asheville : Chiron Publications, [2019] | Includes bibliographical references and index. | Summary: "This work explores the deep archetypal patterns embedded in the African healing initiation, the alchemical opus, and the individuation process through the work of C.G. Jung. The African healer subscribes to dreams the value and meaning that parallels the importance given to dreams in Jungian psychology. As such, this work focuses on the dream and alchemical symbolism within the stages of the African healing initiation, and documents the journey of a Zulu woman's heroic confrontation with her calling to be a healer. The main focus being striving towards wholeness or a transpersonal unity through the direct experience of the unintentional: The numinous "other" with respect to the autonomous reality of the objective psyche, the Self. Here we are offered a return, with consciousness, to the instincts, to an inner numinosity, to the phenomenon of psyche and matter, and spirit in nature. The author's direct and personal collaboration with various indigenous healing communities in South and Southern Africa, Namibia and Botswana provides a rich backdrop to and foundation for her work. The meeting of two cultures in the therapeutic temenos and the ceremonial rituals of the African healing initiation provides the vessel for the transformation necessary for the emergence of something new and as yet largely unarticulated"— Provided by publisher.
Identifiers: LCCN 2019020263 | ISBN 9781630517083 (paperback) | ISBN 9781630517090 (hardcover)
Subjects: LCSH: Traditional medicine—Africa. | Medicine—Africa.
Classification: LCC R651 .R23 2019 | DDC 615.8/8096—dc23
LC record available at https://lccn.loc.gov/2019020263

If the works succeeds, it often works like a miracle . . .
Deo concedente as the alchemists inserted into their recipes.

—C.G. Jung, "The Psychology of the Transference"

Contents

Acknowledgments

Marie-Louise von Franz (1915-1998) was known to comment that when the unconscious supports your creative work, you have an obligation to bring the work into consciousness. I am grateful for the many dreams that accompanied the writing of this work and encouraged me to bring it into a manifest reality.

This work is a testimony to the healers of Lusikisiki in the Eastern Cape, Nyanga, Khayalitsha, Gugeletu, and Da Noon in the Western Cape, Mamelodi, Soweto and Alexandra in Gauteng who unfailingly welcomed me with my white skin, and accepted my often clumsy Western mannerisms, and generously shared many rationally inexplicable phenomena. I remain in awe of their humility, capacity to accept "otherness," and their dedication to their way of life. Mostly, to Ntombi whose courage and clarity I am humbled to have witnessed, and without whom this work would not have been possible.

My sincere thanks to Jennifer Fitzgerald for accepting this work for publication with Chiron and the editorial team for their assistance with the preparation of the manuscript. Thank you to Siobhan Drummond for her initial editorial assistance.

A special thank you to the organisation team of the *Stiftung Jung'sche Psychologie*, Küsnacht, Switzerland, whose support, in part, made the work a reality. My appreciation to the members of the board of the Research and Training Centre for Depth Psychology, Zürich, Switzerland who deepened my knowledge of the work of C.G. Jung and Marie-Louise von Franz, and alchemy in particular.

I am thankful for family, friends and colleagues who believed in the work, with special mention to Hansueli Etter, Charlene Henry, Charles Zeltzer, Mary Stowell, and Robert Mark, and David for his patience and support.

List of Images

Figure 1. *Sangomas* participate in an initiation ceremony

Figure 2. A large multicolored mantis, the theriomorphic form of the creator spirit

Figure 3. Group of healers after an initiation ceremony, Western Cape

Figure 4. A *sangoma* at an initiatory ceremony

Figure 5. An herbalist (*inyanga*) in his apothecary shop in Cape Town, South Africa

Figure 6. An herbalist's apothecary with shelves filled with various indigenous herbs used for healing

Figure 7. A male healer, Eastern Cape, South Africa

Figure 8. A healer dressed in the traditional regalia known as the *amabhayi*

Figure 9. Healer with a cowhide drum

Figure 10. Healers participate in an initiation dance ceremony

Figure 11. Healers participate in ritual *intlombe* ceremony

Figure 12. *Amafahlawana*: ankle bracelets worn during the dance ceremony

Figure 13. Healers dance during the *intlombe*

Figure 14. A *sangoma* drumming at a healing ritual

Figure 15: Two healers dressed in individual regalia

Figure 16: The alchemists at work depicting the different stages of the alchemical process

Figure 17. The four stages of the alchemical process. The four elements are indicated on the balls.

Figure 18. An initiate prepares for the early morning ritual

Figure 19. An aerial view of a traditional Zulu kraal, Kwa-Zulu, Natal

Figure 20. Carved stick used by healers

Figure 21. Black *muthi,* consisting of different indigenous herbs that function as purgatives

Figure 22. An initiate with white face paint and white regalia

Figure 23. Male initiate during the whitening stage

Introduction

Umhlophe, kodwa, Umoya wakho mnyama, ngowase Afrika
You have a white skin, but nonetheless, your spirit belongs to Africa.
—Zulu healer

Despite the early hour, the air is sluggish and thick with heat. It is difficult to breathe. The jeep bounces over the crude roads. The wheels hit a ditch and the cool-drink bottles fall. Outside, frenetic flies intent on every drop of perspiration plague a scattering of lethargic dogs, thin and watchful.

The children run naked in the heat and shout as we make our way carefully over the rugged dirt roads: *"Umlungu, gogo, umlungu,"*— "white people, grandma, white people." She stands hanging her washing and glances at us under hooded eyes, guarded and suspicious. "White people, what do they want now, here today?"

Relief floods her face as we pass her home with the tin roof and cardboard walls. The dust sticks in our throats and clogs our noses. The jeep stops near a dripping tap angled in the permanent mud pool littered with cracked plastic buckets.

It is a Sunday and everyone is at home, sitting on makeshift steps almost on the street. There is little space here. Chicken-wire fences clumsily mark each yard, haphazardly encroaching onto the neighbouring ground.

I climb out of the jeep, shielding my eyes against the harsh and unkind sun, the air visible in the heat. I smile at the old woman collecting water for the morning meal. She avoids my eye.

I am aware of my own conflicting feelings. Even though I can try to talk to you in your tongue, how do I tell you that I do not mean to intrude? My white skin sets me apart.

The entrance to the house is crude. An old steel zinc basin rusts in a corner. The smell of "Sunlight" or "Lifebuoy" soap mixes with the strong, noxious smell of paraffin. The plastic flowers on the table are an incongruous attempt at décor. Posters with *"VIVA ANC"* and *"MANDELA"* cover the walls.

Nozipho, a senior initiate, fills the tiny room, large and powerful. "At last," she breathes, as she clasps me in her buttery arms, "Mama[1] is waiting." Nozipho leads me through the yard and into the largest hut. The inside is dark and refreshingly cool. A strong musky animal smell fills the room. The walls are a rough mud-brick. Crude shelves overflow with glass-bottled tinctures. Animal skins and long plaited strands of herbs hang from rusty nails. After some minutes, Mama Masheba emerges from the curtained-off corner of the room.

Copper bangles and colored beads surround her with a gentle singing sound. She carries a newly made animal-hide drum. She holds the drum out to me. She explains that her ancestors told her in her dream to make this drum for me. I know this is her way of telling me that my presence is accepted. "Today we begin," she smiles, as she ushers us back out into the yard.

We sit for hours. Time seems endless. That true African time that responds not to Western watches, but to a deeper, more ancient flow. The crowd grows. Soon the dusty yard fills with people as if drawn by some mysterious force. There is a curious mix of expectancy in the air. The day warms. Scantily clad children run excitedly through the crowd. Suddenly voices stir the languid air. "Jonas has arrived," says Nozipho. "He is a powerful healer, despite his youth." Jonas is tall and reed thin. His quiet dark face is drawn and gaunt.

The crowd seems to step back. As if by some pre-arranged signal, the voices fall silent and respectful. Jonas acknowledges Nozipho and merely glances at me. He begins to build a fire outside the hut. He works at it for some time. He struggles to start the flames and it seems that the struggle is part of the process.

Finally, the fire takes. Jonas disappears into a small hut. He returns with a small black clay pot.

He places the pot on the fire. "That's the *muthi*, the medicine, for the initiate," Nozipho whispers. Jonas enters the main house and it is some time before he emerges with Mama Masheba. They crawl out of the room on their knees with their hands behind their backs. It looks painful and uncomfortable on the hard stony ground.

Mama Masheba seems to be in a trance. Her face is frozen and her eyes closed. They reach the fire on which the pot is cooking. They each hold a hollow bamboo reed and take turns to draw the *muthi* through the reeds. I am aware of all the expectant faces watching. I realize that I am witnessing the beginning of a journey filled with the inexplicable, yet deeply familiar. I feel a sense of awe and expectation to witness how important this could be: The initiation of a *sangoma*.

The memory is clear and ever present. I was sitting in the hut of an African healer surrounded by the pungent smell of *imphepho*, the indigenous purification herb of the healer, more than 25 years ago. I was aware that I was attracting a good deal of curiosity. The *umlungu*, the white person, was not a common sight in the sacred space of the *sangoma*, the indigenous African healer (Radomsky, 2017).[2] Years later during the analysis of a patient, the meaning of this experience was reflected to me in its opposite. My patient, a Zulu woman, insisted that although her skin was black, it was nothing more than a mask for her white spirit and that she abhorred the rituals and ceremonies of her culture (Radomsky, 2009). She strongly resisted her calling to become initiated into the cultural healing practices of her people. My patient's resistance toward her ancestral calling mirrored my own. To witness the realm of the African healer would require a journey into something simultaneously familiar and foreign with respect to my own culture and race.[3]

I am a white South African. I grew up in the era of the apartheid regime of the old South African government, with its legislated racial segregation and inequality.[4] A time where, in my experience, contact with black people was tinged with mystery, fear, prohibitions, and temptations. It was a world where black people were the nannies, wet nurses, and gardeners in the

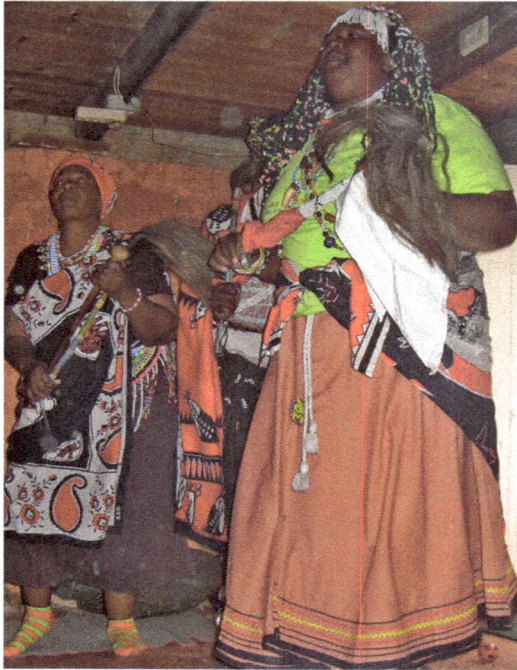

Figure 1: *Sangomas* participate in an initiation ceremony

white homes, entrusted with the care of the children and the home but not considered members of the family.

This was the strange and incongruous space that fascinated me as a young child and instilled awe and incomprehension. I can recall the smells, colors, and strange language that were so foreign to the organized and rational environment of my childhood. This was a place where dreams come alive and ancestral spirits appear in their animal manifestations. Where the serpent, the most powerful of the *amadlozi*, the ancestral spirits, is ever present, and where Mantis, the creator spirit, haunts the night skies. As such, when my dreams seemed to demand that I give attention to this realm, it was both natural and terrifying.

Initially, I was slow to respond, to make sense of the dreams or to hear their voices. I spent many years shrugging them off. Others found them fascinating, but they filled me with fear, a foreboding, and an overwhelming sense of responsibility. In my ignorance or inflation, I pretended that by ignoring them they would go elsewhere. However, dreams walk a larger

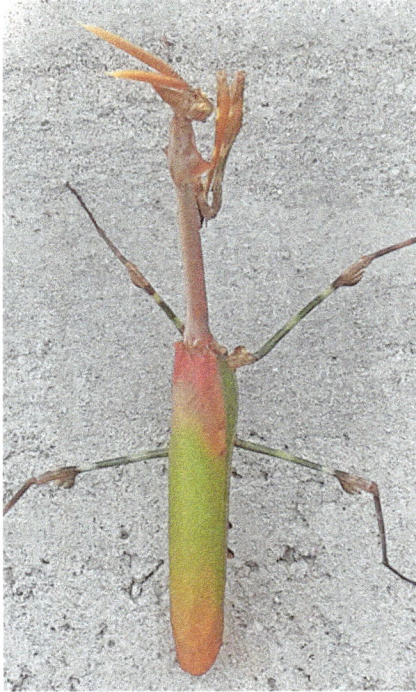

Figure 2. As I sat writing these words, this large multicolored mantis, a theriomorphic form of the creator spirit, flew through the open window and landed on the wall near my writing desk

space than I could begin to conjure. As a depth psychologist with a focus on the psychology of C.G. Jung, I had long given credence to the importance of dreams. I shared these dreams with an African friend who spoke of the connection between the dreams and the *thwasa*, the initiate in his tradition. "They are not just going to go away," he cautioned. "Once the dreams come, you must listen."

When Mama Masheba, a healer with whom I would work closely, appeared suddenly in my life in the 1980s, the risk to her and to me was considerable. Mama Masheba had come to tell me her ancestors had revealed to her in her dreams the white woman whom she was to teach about her traditions. She expressed her awareness that her presence would be difficult for me to understand and accept, and that she was not in a hurry. Her serene dark face reflected both her certainty and my uncertainty. She said she would wait while the Western part of me battled with a far older knowledge. My acceptance of her presence, while disconcerting, was not unexpected, as I had seen her arrival in my own dreams.

Thus began my long and challenging discovery of the realm of African healing. A journey that equipped me to be able to reflect, years later, the conflict in my patient and would allow me to hold both the culture she aspired to, which my white Western skin represented, and the culture that was her ancestral heritage.[5]

The analysis of my patient, whom I will call Ntombi,[6] straddled a period of four years. During this time, Ntombi slowly came to embrace her cultural heritage and to engage in her own initiation into the African healing realm. Her analysis in the urban setting of my practice was interspersed with initiatory ceremonies and rituals held at her rural birthplace in KwaZulu Natal.

As the seemingly disparate processes of Ntombi's analysis and her initiation evolved, I became aware, first and foremost, of the theme of opposites that wove a tapestry between these two worlds. In the outer collective, South Africa, the gene pool of humankind, is a land where opposites are visible and vacillate between depth of creativity and disregard for life. Throughout the ages, Africa has captured the imagination of many, drawing them hypnotically to the land of the first people and wild beasts. Day to day, one is faced with extreme polarities: hot and cold, drought and floods, wealth and poverty, humanitarianism and extreme abuse of human rights, peace and violence, geological beauty and devastation, and most obviously, black and white. The tip of Africa is where the two oceans meet, the warm Indian and the cold Atlantic.

South Africa is pollinated with diverse and conflicting ideologies that manifest in a number of challenges for living. Jung (1977) observed that Africa "offers a spirit of greater openness to the unconscious, increased attention to dreams, a sharper sense of the totality of the physical and the psychic . . . a livelier taste for self-knowledge" (p. 399). Psychologically, the faculties of thinking, feeling, sensation, and intuition, in both their extraverted and introverted attitudes, are simultaneously challenged.

South Africa has a complex demographic marked by a heterogeneous population base as a result of socio-political issues brought on by colonialism, the legacy of apartheid, divisions within ethnic groups, and migration (see appendix 1). Working in South Africa, it is, in my experience, incumbent upon the analyst to develop a relationship with the historical development and cultural phenomena and to navigate the infinitely delicate and complex terrain of race, prejudice, privilege, oppression, and humanity.

The release of Nelson Mandela in 1990 signaled the beginning of the transition toward a democracy. The rainbow notion was born. This term, coined by Archbishop Desmond Tutu, was intended to encapsulate the unity of multiculturalism in a country once defined by the strict divisions of black and white. Recently, this largely naïve image has been tainted by the realities of a nation in transition.

Marie-Louise von Franz (1999a) explained that the acceptance of new political parties that seem to offer new beginnings is the effect of the projection onto the new party for a renewal. But when this transformation is not internalized and is only externally projected, it usually becomes negative.

South Africa today is a maturing democracy 24 years old and the embodiment of an emerging adolescent collective consciousness. Intense and poetic, molded by rebellion, passion, hubris and idealism, it is a developing democracy that strives for independence through the search for an identity and the discovery of a new myth. When interviewed in the film *Matter of Heart,* Jung reflected that "man has always lived with a myth and we think that we are able to be born today and to live in no myth, without history. This is a disease. Man is only complete when he has a relationship to history" (Whitney, 1986).

For the individual, South Africa can be experienced as a land of shadow that challenges one to embrace this aspect. The concept of the shadow is pivotal to Jung's psychology, which he defined as "the thing [a person] has no wish to be" (1946b, para. 470). The shadow aspects are thus often projected onto the other by the individual manifesting in envy, exclusion, preconception, and rejection of "otherness." In the outer collective, shadow projections are latent in divisions in a society, including prejudice, racism, totalitarianism, discrimination, intolerance, judgment and partiality. As Jung (1946a) cautioned with respect to the shadow projection:

> The underestimation of [this] psychological factor is likely to take a bitter revenge. It is therefore high time we caught up with ourselves in this matter. . . . because self-knowledge . . . is preoccupied with the psychological shadow, which is normally denied . . . The task that faces our age is indeed almost insuperably

difficult. It makes the highest demands on our responsibilities if we are not to be guilty of another *trahison des clercs*. (para. 569)

As I reflect on the future of the multilayered complexity of Africa, often oversimplified and misunderstood, I was reminded of Jung's words as reported by Barbara Hannah. When Jung was asked about his prognosis for humanity, he replied: "I think it depends on how many people can stand the tension of opposites in themselves. If enough can, I think we shall escape the worst" (in Hannah, 1981, p. 8). Jung is referring to the psychological truth that when the conflict of opposites remains unconscious in the individual, this conflict is projected outwardly onto others and society as a whole. This seems applicable to the collective South African psyche, and to Ntombi in particular, who as an individual was called to become conscious of the tension of opposites in her psyche and the development of a new personal myth.

Against this background, I began to catch a glimmer of the parallels between the African initiatory rites and the psychology of C.G. Jung during the work with Ntombi. These parallels included the inner topography of the unconscious psyche mirrored in the primary attention given to dreams within both realms and the stages of the alchemical opus as described by Jung. Both focus on the transformation in the inner world. Both embody the archetypal images nascent in the objective psyche.

As the impetus for this work was born and the impulse to share its wisdom became urgent, I had the following dream:

I am lying on a mat covered with skins in a hut. The hut is a typical African healer's reed and mud hut found in rural Africa. I can smell the pungent aroma of imphepho burning. Sitting on my left is an African woman, a healer. Her dark skin is ageless, yet she seems ancient. She has been waiting for me to awaken. She brings me a bowl of healing herbs and oils and rubs the oils into my skin. To my right I can hear the drums. There is a male healer drumming. I feel a sense of peace and surrender. The woman goes away and returns carrying some photos. She lays them down on the mat in front of me. They are black-and-white photos of Jung. She collects the photos, smiles, and gives them to me.

Encouraged by this dream and many others, I was able to continue with the work.

The amplification of the rich symbolic world of the African healer offers us a glimpse into a living system from which to begin to unravel the great mysteries of life, death, and the afterlife. We are further offered a return, with consciousness, to the instincts, to an inner numinosity, to the phenomenon of psyche and matter, and spirit in nature. Here we enter the realms of the unfathomable mystery of the unitary nature of spirit and matter. In this realm, synchronistic phenomena demand the realization that matter transgresses into the realm of sprit and spirit transgresses into the realm of matter.

It is my hope that by describing the cosmology of the African healer—the phenomenon of the ancestors, the living dead, the ceremonies, rituals, and practices—that we, too, in our limited capacity, may begin to catch a glimpse of this eternal mystery. By association, this would embrace a return to the fecund, the feminine principle, the earth, instinct, and the body, all of which have been neglected in the pursuit of the sometimes one-sided rational consciousness that characterizes the Western zeitgeist, often resulting in a multitude of neuroses.

This includes documenting the initiatory process and how such experiences look in reality when there is a serious attempt to grasp the unknown realms of the soul. Such attempts, within the African healing realm—as it is with the alchemical opus—have numerous variations based on individual and collective differences, but nonetheless are primordial images of a universal archetypal pattern.

This work is thus a response, in part, to the unconscious urges that seemed to demand some concrete manifestation, to the numerous requests over many years from the healers to document and to tell their stories, and to my patient Ntombi, whose permission made such a work possible. A further impetus for this work is the relationship of the individuation process relative to the fate of humanity in the coming Aion of the Aquarian age. Von Franz (1998) noted that "the task of man in the Aquarian age is to become conscious of his larger inner presence, the anthropos, and to give the utmost care to nature instead of exploiting it" (p. 136). This seems to be most pertinent given the current global socio-political, cultural, economic and climatic turbulence.

The main focus here is to document one woman's journey back to her origins, and as such, reflect an image of the individuation process mirrored in the stages of an initiation. I have chosen the presentation of a single case specifically because this allows for the focused portrayal of a journey that bridged two seemingly opposing epistemologies within an individual. Again the importance of the inner process of the individual in the coming Aion is emphasized by Jung (1951) when he stated that "Aquarius will constellate the problem of the union of opposites. . . . This problem can be solved . . . only by the individual . . . via his experience of the living spirit" (para. 142). In this way, we are offered a unique window into the realm of opposites and how these are potentially integrated through a respectful attitude to the unconscious psyche. As Jung (1934b) noted:

> In the last analysis, the essential thing is the life of the individual. This alone makes history, here alone do the great transformations take place, and the whole future, the whole history of the world, ultimately springs from these hidden sources in individuals. (para. 315)

I remain cautious about the sharing information about sacred rituals, and I am aware that such secret knowledge must be approached with care. Initiatory phenomena are "mysterious things," which cannot be easily explained and require an acceptance of the unitary nature of the conscious mind and the unconscious psyche. I once asked an old healer what he thought about my writing of "such things" and if I was in some way profaning spirit. He laughed at me and asked me in turn if I really thought that I could in any way profane spirit by anything I did on a human level. His easy wisdom pulled me down out of my inflation. His response reflected his awareness that in his belief system spiritual knowledge can be described to all. He buffered his awareness with the warning that where potential danger lies is in trying to experience these mysteries without an authentic call from the Self. As such, I have been mindful of his wisdom. I am deeply aware that much must be left unsaid. I would encourage each reader to be open to initiatory phenomena that they are individually called to embrace, and which take many different forms, embedded in a myriad of life experiences, including that of depth analysis.

My discussion of sacred information, ceremonies and dreams of Ntombi, will be limited to those related to the rituals that are mostly performed as part of the public domain, that have echoes and reflections in the healing ceremonies of the African traditions. The dreams presented in this work were selected from numerous dreams and focus specifically on those that are pertinent to the stages of Ntombi's initiation. I do not make any claims of generalization to the entire system of African healing. The African healing system is based almost exclusively on an oral tradition. The shape that an initiation takes is governed by individual requirements guided by dreams and ancestral communications. There is no unitary perspective with respect to the African healing realm due to the disparate and distinct tribal communities within the vast multicultural continent that is Africa. The documentation of Ntombi's journey, thus, cannot be construed as a formula for initiation or a model for therapeutic intervention.

My aim is to stay true to the cosmology and culture of the material presented. Where relevant and applicable, I will draw on amplifications from the alchemical opus explored by Jung. While it is not possible to provide a complete discussion of alchemical images and symbols, my hope is to present aspects of the alchemical stages as archetypal phenomena that arise spontaneously in the unconscious when there is a serious attempt to engage with the autonomous psyche. These archetypal phenomena are indicative of patterns of transformation and healing. As such there is a close connection between alchemy, the African healing initiation, and the psychology of the unconscious. As Jung (1946b) explained, "alchemy describes . . . the same psychological phenomenology which can be observed in the analysis of unconscious processes" (para. 399). I hope to demonstrate how an ancient alchemical process is alive and well in a modern lived experience, and how the inner psychic processes of initiation rites are, in turn, an alchemical opus.

The analysis of Ntombi accompanied her during her initiation into her own cultural legacy, supporting and encouraging the development of an enlivening and vitalizing relationship to and with the unconscious. Her process was guided by her dreams and exhibits individual aspects that may not be identical to any other. In some small way, this demonstrates the autonomy and objectivity of deep psychic processes. The meeting of two cultures in the therapeutic temenos potentially provided the vessel for

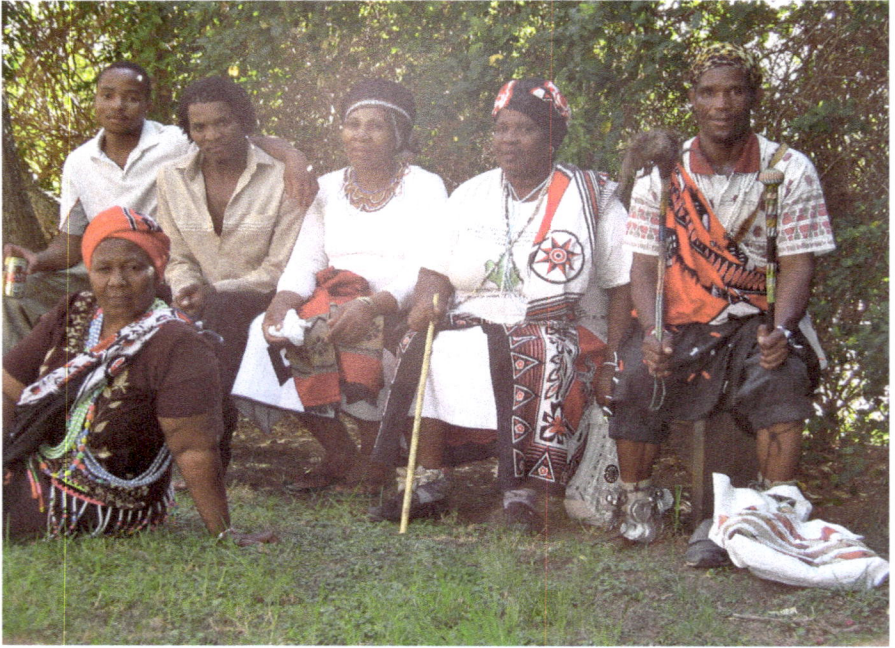

Figure 3. A group of healers after an initiation ceremony, Western Cape

transformation and for the emergence of something new, and as yet largely unarticulated.

I will attempt to hold such a work as an aspect of the creative individuation process, or an image of the archetype of individuation, which by definition remains incomplete and unknowable. Jung (1955-56) taught that the immediate goal of individuation is to nurture a conscious relationship with the Self through "the experience and production of the symbol of the totality" (para. 770). As such, my aim is to illustrate the transformation of the individual through the initiation into the healer and a connection to an inner numinous God-image.[7] Essentially, what I hope to convey is a reflection of Jung's main premise: that of the reality and autonomy of the unconscious psyche. The following anecdote reminded me of the healer's relationship to the psyche and their awareness of the attitude and position required by the ego in this relationship:

INTRODUCTION

Some years back I was invited to attend an initiation ceremony in the rural Eastern Cape. We had all risen early before sunrise. It was a cold and wet winter morning, the ground still frozen from the night's frost. I dressed and went out to join the group gathered to welcome the new initiate. Because I was cold, I wore my shoes and socks. It did not take long before I was approached by an old healer. She stood stoically in front of me, her wizened face a mask of disapproval. Silently, she stared at my feet, placing her own gnarled bare foot next to my shoes. Her meaning was clear: This is sacred ground that you are desecrating with your shoes. I immediately retreated, duly chastised, to remove my shoes and to bear the cold.

Chapter 1
Lokuzalwa:
The Birth of a Healer

This sickness is really a soul sickness.
—Ntombi

Ntombi came to see me in my practice in a state of despair. She reported crippling anxiety and fear, difficulties sleeping and concentrating, mood shifts, loss of appetite, and weight changes. She seemed to satisfy the criteria necessary for the diagnosis of clinical depression. She had already consulted a Western-trained psychiatrist, who was treating her for a major depressive disorder with a pharmacological regime, in accordance with the *Diagnostic and Statistical Manual of Mental Disorders* (DSM), but with little effect.

Ntombi explained that she had come to see me as a last resort, as she had heard that I had some understanding of her culture and that I worked with dreams. She said that she needed me to stop the dreams, to make them go away. As I was white, she wanted me to help her extract herself from the traditional ways of her people. She was at the time in her final year as a medical student, living with her white boyfriend, and she had just received a sponsorship to work and study further in a northern European country. She was adamant that this was the fulfilment of her life's purpose.

I reflected at the time that her life's journey seemed to be flowing in accordance with her needs. She appeared crestfallen and somewhat fearful. She replied:

Yes, it is, very much. I seem to have everything I want on the surface. I should be happy. It's just . . . well, the dreams they worry me. I don't want to sleep anymore, I cannot stand the dreams. I make sure that I am so exhausted at night, perhaps I won't dream.

The dreams were causing obvious distress for Ntombi. I was concerned in that I had in mind C.G. Jung's idea of the capacity for dreams to renew a dry, stagnant state of mind or as the moisture that enlivens the unconscious (1955–56, para. 190). Jung noted that "if you prove receptive to this 'call of the wild,' the longing for fulfilment will quicken the sterile wilderness of your soul as rain quickens the dry earth." However, before we could explore the meaning of the dreams for Ntombi, I inquired in the anamnesis about her background and her family.

Ntombi had been born into a rural Zulu family in a small village on the outskirts of KwaZulu-Natal, on the east coast of South Africa, during the apartheid era. Growing up, she was exposed to racial discrimination that resulted in extremes of poverty, malnutrition, and poor education and health care. As a result of urbanization and her family's need to find work, she moved to the city townships as a young girl.

Ntombi had quickly assessed the urban life as offering opportunities, sophistication, and the promise of wealth, helping her escape from her oppressed existence. At the same time, she came to devalue and despise what she called "that primitiveness" of her ancestral home and lifestyle. When I enquired about her family in the rural areas, she told me that her grandfather was a well-respected African healer in her home village. He died recently, but she had not gone back for the burial. Within the Zulu culture, as it is for many cultures, the burial of a close family member is an important occasion. As her grandfather was the village healer, he would have been honored in death and given a ceremonial burial. A granddaughter not attending the funeral would be considered a great slight on the family name.

Ntombi felt she needed to have all that city life could offer her, and this was in direct contradiction to the values that her grandparents upheld. She resisted going to visit the homestead, her place of origin. She had slowly transformed her appearance to reflect the images and values of the white culture that she prized. She had, over the years, used very dangerous skin lightening products, as well as adopting a style of dress that was the antithesis of her African culture.

Reinforced by her parents, who had adopted the Christian religion of the white people and in so doing rejected their traditional African practices as heretical, Ntombi had grown up praying to the "white" god embedded in the white religious dogma. Ntombi's adoption of the white Christian religion seemed to me to reflect a dogmatic form of the religious experience in that she had lost the true religious connection that could provide numinous meaning in life.

At the time, and still today, very few white people were conversant in any of the African languages, and African people who depended on whites for employment typically chose anglicized names to make it easier for their white employers. Ntombi had thus introduced herself to me using her Western English name, and she was surprised when I asked for her Zulu birth name. The meaning of names in Zulu culture reflect Jung's words when he observed that

> the name of the individual is his soul, and hence the custom of using the ancestor's name to reincarnate the ancestral soul in the new-born child. This means nothing less than that the ego consciousness is recognized as being an expression of the soul. (1934a, para. 665)

In post-apartheid South Africa, and in Ntombi's projected experiences, "whiteness" is often still prized and aligned with a Westernized way of being, a standard against which she measured her self-acceptance and self-worth. While racism is no longer a legislated concept, race often remains a primary point of reference. Racial messages are still conveyed through symbolic projections attached to whiteness and blackness. Whiteness is often about economic success, wealth, intellectual superiority, orderliness, and rationality. Blackness is about chaos, violence, crime, and the irrational.

Von Franz (1997a) noted that whenever the historic-religious mythology of a people is destroyed, the people lose their feeling of belonging to a meaningful whole and become disoriented. In apartheid South Africa, for many of the black people, cultural mythology was outlawed and with it the feeling for meaning in existence. Materialism replaced spiritual and cultural values.

Ntombi was training to become a Western-based allopathic medical practitioner, with the associated potential accumulation of material wealth, recognition, and prestige, located firmly within the deterministic and reductive biomedical model of sickness and health. At the time, for a black

29

woman to study medicine in South Africa was fraught with discriminations and prejudice. Nonetheless, Ntombi embraced her studies as her ticket out of her ethnic classification as well as her insurance against the poverty and deprivation of her childhood. She had faced many hardships in order to gain a secondary education as well as entry into a medical training program, and as a result she was nearing midlife at the time of her analysis.

From my first contact with her, it appeared that Ntombi's greatest fear was that her symptoms were not in fact those of a psychiatrically classifiable disorder, but perhaps indications of a calling from her cultural heritage, and psychologically, an encounter with the Self. The African healing cosmology thus confronted her with an alternative that she could not yet entertain. Her cultural cosmology presented a challenge to the Westernized view of reality that she had acquired.

For Ntombi, to embrace a heritage that she had chosen to reject would mean giving up "all she had worked for" with respect to her need to adopt a Westernized way of being. For her, this symbolized a regression and a failure of integration. Her symptoms took the form of repeated suicidal ideation in that she often expressed, in her desperation, "I would rather die than face this."

Ntombi's initial emotional state was one of dehumanization and isolation. She described feelings of alienation and helplessness, and she seemed to embody Jung's (1961b) image of feeling

> isolated in the cosmos . . . no longer involved in nature . . . Thunder is no longer the voice of god, nor is lightning his avenging missile. No river contains a spirit, no tree means a man's life, no snake is the embodiment of wisdom and no mountain harbours a great demon. Neither do things speak to him nor can he speak to things, like stones, springs, plants and animals. He no longer has a bush soul identifying him with a wild animal . . . and the emotional energy it generated has sunk into the unconscious. (para. 585)

What was required of Ntombi seemed to be what is required in the individuation process, that of a shift toward an individual psychology and away from the collective psychology. This entailed letting go of the acquired collective doctrines of the church religion and a transition to an individual experience of the numinosity of the Self. Faced with the upsurge of the irrational and feelings of disorientation, as well as the fear of losing herself,

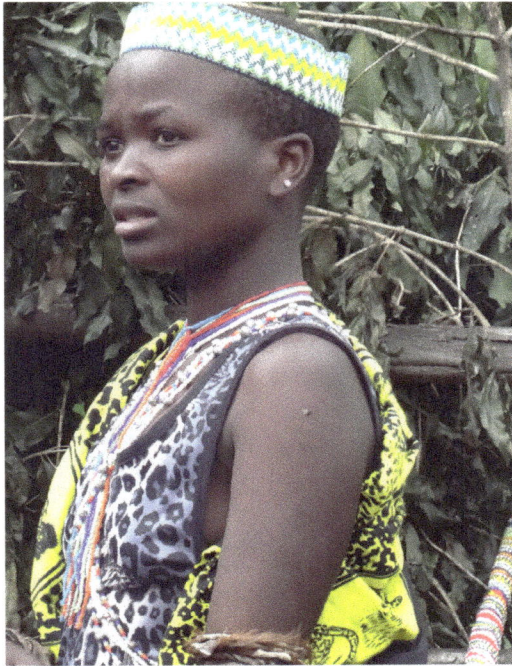

Figure 4. A *sangoma* at an initiation ceremony

Ntombi's challenge in relating to her inner conflict required a confrontation with her usual conscious attitude. Such a confrontation called for a plasticity of the ego and had to allow for the inclusion of inconsistencies and doubt, which in turn herald the possibility for change. In the collective, this challenge is reflected in the daily reminders of the vacillation between opposites embodied in the themes of "black" and "white."

It is from this atmosphere that my patient emerged and in which she struggled with her own individual attempt at reconciliation. This transformation was embedded in the phenomenon of the initiation process and the world of the Zulu healing cosmology.

Cosmology of the African Healer

Existing literature about the cosmology of the African healing phenomenon is meager. Researchers note that early white settlers described the healers as "charismatic charlatans coercing others through clever manipulations of

31

esoteric knowledge and granted inappropriate worth by a credulous and anxiety ridden people" (Peek, 1991, p. 3). Sadly, this prejudice is still prevalent today with respect to the indigenous healing traditions and rituals.

This cosmology presents a challenge to Western predilections and view of reality. In academic circles, Western-based scientific paradigms often still predominate. The Western mind dissects, dissolves, and differentiates. The African mind when it looks at the arrangement of things or events accepts it as it is and seeks instead the meaning in the events. When indigenous epistemologies, based largely on oral tradition, are expressed that perhaps have not been subjected to the rigors of so-called evidence-based methodologies, they risk being dismissed as unfounded.

Jung (1961a) commented that his experience with Native Americans made him aware of his "imprisonment in the cultural consciousness of the white man" (p. 247). He maintained that the beliefs and practices of indigenous peoples served the function of making their lives cosmologically meaningful. Whereas for Westerners who predominantly use reason to formulate the meaning of life, Jung noted that "knowledge does not enrich us, it removes us more and more from the mythic world, in which we were once at home, by right of birth" (1961a, p. 252).

In the outer collective, the main aim of indigenous peoples is the survival of the group and healthy social functioning. Here the importance of the individual resides largely in his or her service to the group. The different value given to the individual versus the collective is a crucial concept that underlies the African healing system. Healing is often public and requires the participation of the community. Certain healing ceremonies cannot be held without the presence of the individual patient's family, who are required to fulfill a number of obligations. It is too easy to interpret this process as undifferentiated, stuck in the collective, or as a regressive descent into unconsciousness. To see the African psyche as pre-logical is to miss the essence of the African epistemology with an integrated view of psyche, soul, and nature. Rather the relationship between the individual and the collective functions to nurture a living vein between the individual, the ancestors (psychologically, the collective unconscious), and collective consciousness. As von Franz reminded us, "we have to revive the idea of soul in matter" (in Rossi, 2008, p. 151).

In my experience working and collaborating with healers over many years, I have come to understand the process as a difference in the focus of psychic resources, a difference in the underlying assumptions that reflect an internal logic. That is, for me, the African healing ceremonies and practices can perhaps be understood psychologically as the preservation of the dialogue between the conscious ego, the Self, and the collective un-conscious. The goal of the initiatory process for the healer embodies individuation imagery and experiences of immense numinosity, and transformational effect.

Illness and Healing in the African Worldview

The African healer does not categorize ill health into physical and psychological aspects. Rather the healer, as noted by Mircea Eliade (1972), participates in the world in a meaningful way, surrounded by the sacred. For the healer, illness often reflects a disharmony with the spirit world and treatment involves the development of a relationship to the illness in order to restore harmony, which in turn affects the "cure." A healer commented:

> It is not just a body problem; it is also a spiritual problem. If the spirit is not right the illness will return or come again as another illness. Body, mind, and spirit are connected; it is not enough to only heal the body or the spirit. We have to treat the spiritual energy as well and that involves the ancestors. But people need to be helped to help themselves. If they do not participate in their healing, no one can help them.[8]

The biomedical world strives to eradicate illness and as such the doctor stands in a kind of "opposition" to the symptoms, with little attention given to the symbolic meaning of symptoms. Whereas in the indigenous healing system symptoms of illness are often regarded as a direct communication from the ancestors, an indication that something is out of balance on a spiritual level. Psychologically, this would be akin to understanding the symbolic meaning embedded in the physical symptoms. The ancestors form the core of the connectedness of the healer to the sacred and to the healing. The healer mediates the healing of the patient through the collaboration with these divine powers imbued with numinous energy. As a healer explained:

When someone comes to see me, for all types of problems like physical, emotional, anything. They come in and sit down. We do not need to talk. I sit and burn some herbs and go into a trance. The ancestors speak to me or through me and tell the person what is wrong and what they need to do to get well or to restore the harmony. Sometimes it's a sacrifice, sometimes other things. But always the ancestors are respected and thanked.

There are different types of African healers, each with their own specializations, knowledge, and expertise. There are also diverse terms used to describe the different healer types. For the purposes of this work, I will focus on the terminology most often used colloquially. The herbalist is known as the *inyanga*. The *sanuzi* is the prophet or diviner. The *sangoma* is a Zulu healer who is both diviner and herbalist. Healers are also referred to as "traditional," "indigenous," or "African." The term *shaman* is not commonly used in South Africa. In addition, *witch doctor* is considered a pejorative term, largely as a result of white colonists who vilified indigenous practices. The material is this book focuses almost exclusively on the initiation of the *sangoma*, the Zulu healer.

More than 85 percent of black people will consult an African or indigenous healer before consulting a Western medical doctor. Very few medical practitioners recognize the effectiveness of the indigenous healing practices. The healers, however, will also identify symptoms of illness that require a medical intervention, and they will send patients to Western doctors for treatment.

Within the category of the *sangoma*, it is possible to differentiate between two broad pathways to becoming a healer. The more traditional pathway is identified by a calling and mediated by elder healers (see chapter 4). This process most closely resembles that of the medicine man or medicine woman found in other indigenous systems. The less common initiation is one in which the initiate undergoes a process in direct relationship with the sacred (see chapter 9). This more closely resembles the shamanic traditions of North and South America, Siberia, and other places. Within the Zulu culture these two pathways are not necessarily exclusive. The initiate may undergo both types of initiations depending on what is called for by the sacred or the ancestors.

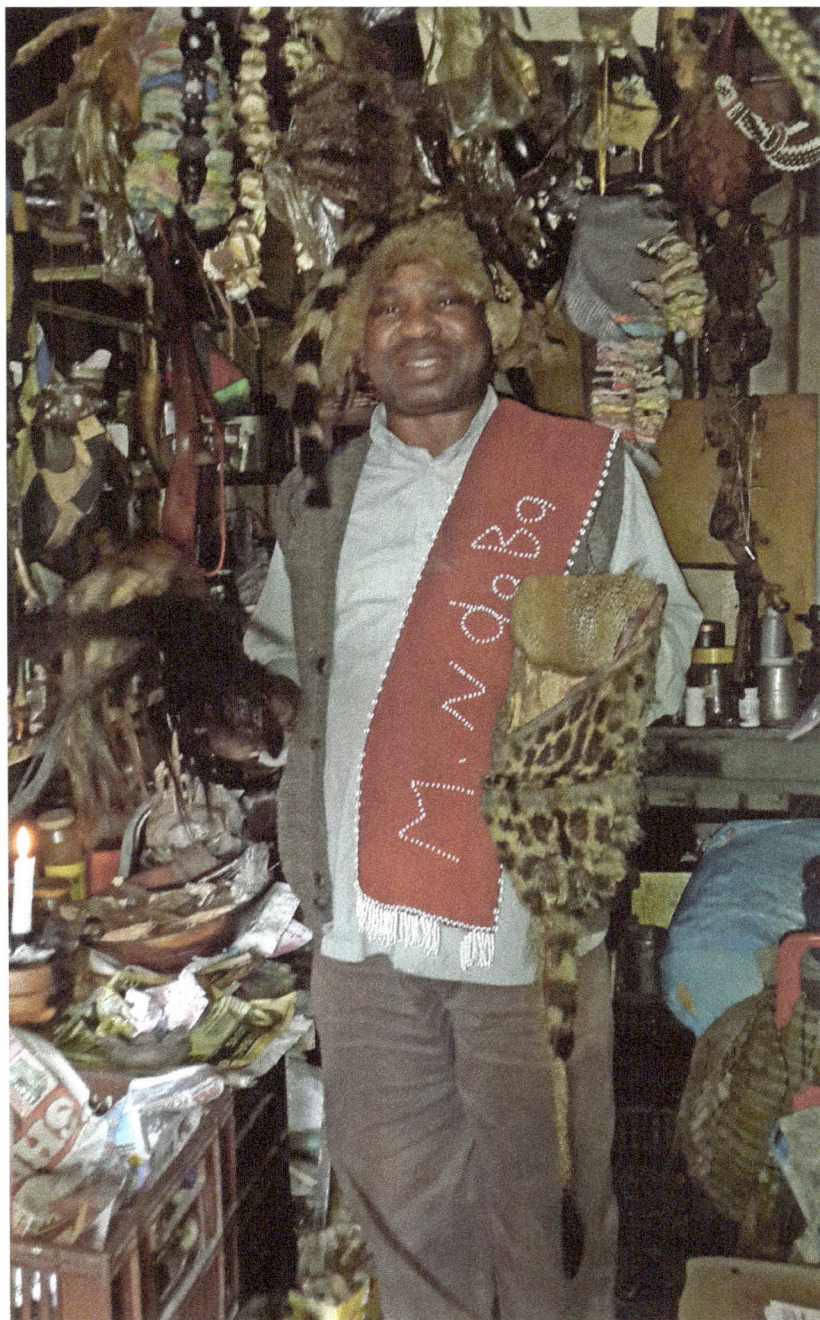

Figure 5. An herbalist (*inyanga*) in his apothecary shop in Cape Town, South Africa

In both initiations, the neophyte undergoes a transformation and emerges with healing knowledge. A difference between these two types of initiations resides in the way healing transpires. In the former, healing involves complex rituals and a variety of remedies or *muthi* (herbal medicines). In the latter, the healer's primary role is that of incorporating the illness into his or her own being where it is transformed through the restoration of harmony with the ancestors, or from a psychological understanding, to be in harmony with the Self.

The overriding factor in both systems is that healing is essentially a spiritual process. The primary purpose of the healer is to maintain a harmony with the spirit world, and the loss of life is not always considered discordant with this concept. Rather, the loss of soul is the gravest of occurrences, which results in the loss of meaning in life. For the African healer, the purpose of life is spiritual development. The healer conceives of health as knowing life and death as aspects of a totality. Jung (1934a) noted that to the indigenous person:

> the psyche appears as the source of life . . . which has objective reality. [He] knows how to converse with his soul; it becomes vocal within him because it is not simply he himself and his consciousness. To primitive man the psyche is not (as it is to us), the epitome of all that is subjective and subject to will; on the contrary, it is something objective, self-subsistent, and living its own life. (para. 666)[9]

Jung (1975) takes this idea further:

> People speak of *belief* when they have lost *knowledge*. Belief and disbelief are god surrogates. The naïve primitive does not *believe*, he *knows* because the inner experience rightly means as much to him as the outer . . . He lives in *one* world where as we live in only one half and merely believe in the other or not at all. (p. 5)

A largely rational approach, reliant on the thinking function, promotes one-sidedness. This characterizes the premise of evidence-based medical epistemologies and in turn removes us from our inherent nature and any concept of an inner and outer whole or unity. The instinctual or material body has increasingly come to be regarded as less relevant in the rational world dominated by the masculine logos principle, as it represents the lower, animal aspect in conjunction with the feminine, the fecund, and the Eros principle. It seems to me that what we can learn from the African healing realm is the redemption of the feminine, the instinct and the body, with a conscious return to what Jung (1977) advised in mitigation of this one-sidedness in order "to halt the fatal dissociation that exits between man's higher and lower being" (p. 396). This "fatal dissociation" seems to be commonplace today, and at times, in my experience, even reflects how some aspects of Jung's psychology are interpreted today. Many patients in my consulting room express a deep dissatisfaction with conventional religious and medical practices. This has resulted in the search for alternative experiences of the sacred. The shadow aspect of this search, when it is undifferentiated or unconscious emerges in the burgeoning of false initiations and pseudo-spiritual programs.

Effectiveness of the African Healing Initiation Procedures

The general structure of the initiation process is recognizable across most different tribal initiations. During this rigorous and demanding time, the initiate acquires knowledge about herbal remedies, rituals, and dream interpretation. Most importantly, from a psychological understanding, the initiate undergoes a process of self-development and maturation wherein she or he is expected to integrate previously unacknowledged and unknown parts of the personality and to develop an accord with inner aspects.

The aim is to develop the ego strength of the initiate to help him or her withstand the constant brooding of the ancestors without becoming disturbed, to integrate powerful forces of the unconscious, and to avoid dangerous inflations. Through the initiation, the deeper levels of the unconscious that have been activated during the process, and which initially caused distress for the initiate, are integrated as meaningful manifestations of the psyche.

In psychological language, this is the process whereby the ego is confronted with the Self and the need to pay attention to the messages from the unconscious. Providing the process is followed carefully and faithfully, something is birthed, a new symbol of the Self in the form of the healer, symbolic perhaps of an image of an individuated personality with a greater

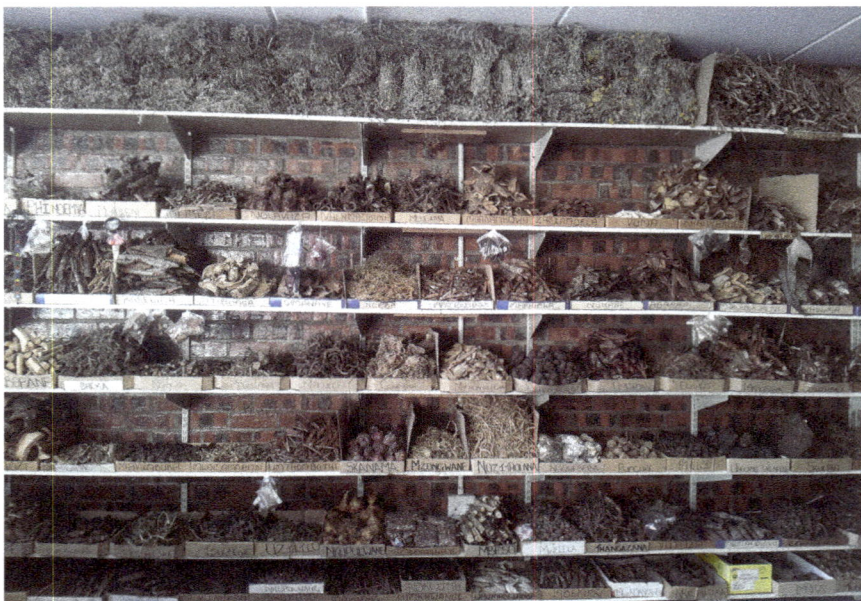

Figure 6. An herbalist's apothecary with shelves filled with various indigenous herbs used for healing

consciousness and responsibility, marked by courage, humility, and a knowledge of history, serving the sacred both inner and outer. In the words of a healer:

> At first I was terrified . . . but after I accepted the calling, every-thing went fine. I started like an infant and then I progressed onwards as my abilities grew with each stage. The illness goes away once you accept the calling. I am now a healer . . . it gives me peace of mind. It opens things for me. But is also very difficult. People reject you because you seem to know too much. They fear you so I learnt to be quiet, unless they come to consult me. Then I will tell them.

The effectiveness of the initiation healing procedures is based on two fundamental aspects: First, the acceptance of the calling is understood as a service to the ancestors. The attitude of the initiate to the unconscious material is one of humility, reverence, and respect. Second, the healer-initiate dyad is of utmost importance, and a symbiotic relationship develops not only on the conscious level but between respective ancestors as well, that is, on the unconscious level. The ancestors of the healer communicate with the ancestors of the initiate, thereby circumventing ego-consciousness and all the barriers and resistances that go with it.

The quintessence of the initiation illustrates the psychological truth, as noted by Edward Edinger (1972), that "the experience of the Self in the individuation process conveys to the ego . . . qualities that result from increasing awareness and relationship to the transpersonal . . . dimension of the psyche" (p. 266). It is this relationship that was embodied in both the analytical and initiatory experiences of Ntombi. The prominence given to dreams in both Jungian psychology and the realm of the African healer underlies this relationship.

The Central Role of Dreams

Dreams occupy a crucial place in the initiatory process as well as in the Zulu healing cosmology. Akin to Jung's dictum that the central problem of analytical treatment is dream analysis, echoed through the ages and hallowed in time as the means by which God communicates with man. It is through the medium of dreams that those who listen hear God's song, as Psalm 127 reflects: "for He giveth unto His beloved in their sleep."

The documented importance of dreams for the purposes of healing proliferate the ancient world, including Greece, the Middle East, Rome, Egypt, and India. Illness and dreams were communications from the gods and thus approached with reverence, numinosity, and dignity. Patients came to the healing centers of Asclepius with physical illnesses as well as troubled minds. Hippocrates acknowledged the numinosity of dreams through which the otherwise unknowable becomes known. C.A. Meier (1989) noted that music, singing, dance, and ritual cleansings were used as healing aids and to induce a receptive frame of mind to stimulate dreaming. According to Jung (1940) "every dream . . . carries a message. It not only tells you that something is amiss in the depths of your being, it also brings you a solution for getting out of the crisis" (para. 32).

For the African healer, dreams are the communications from the ancestors that function to awaken the dreamer to certain attitudes or practices in daily life that are out of balance with the ancestral needs. The ancestors, through dreams and visions, are said to guide, encourage, and prepare the initiate for further development. The dreams of the initiates are thus diagnostic and prognostic as well as outlining treatment requirements and thus differ from initiate to initiate depending on individual needs and individual levels of awareness and development. These inner stirrings and voices compel the dreamer to take note and to bring into conscious life the changes required. Serious illness is the outcome of the risk of neglecting these messages. Jung (1948b) discussed the nature of dreams and noted that "the dream does in fact concern itself with both health and sickness . . . this has often proved helpful . . . where the differential diagnosis between organic and psychogenic symptoms presented difficulties" (para. 531). As a healer explained:

> We never dismiss our dreams. We are aware that there is a message behind the dreams. There are different many different meanings in the dreams as well as symbols. In dreams we will find the voice of the ancestors. In the dreams these voices come alive. It is a bit like a puzzle or a treasure hunt.

The Zulu word for dream is *ipupo,* which also implies "to fly," and the word for sleep is *butongo,* which implies "to be with the gods or ancestors." Thus sleeping and dreaming take on a primary importance as to sleep is to fly with the gods. The absence of dreams is a cause for distress and interpreted as a sign of displeasure from the ancestors. During the initiation and training of the initiate, the dreams function to structure the process as well as to inform the different rituals that are needed. The dream will also indicate when the initiate is ready to proceed further in the training or to function independently. The qualified healer will also be informed by his or her own dreams about the initiate.

Types of Dreams

The dreams within the African healing epistemology are divided into big and small dreams. The small dreams, *amaphupho amancane*, are for personal use only and indicate minor changes that are necessary in the individual's daily life. The big dreams, *amaphupho amakhulu*, carry ancestral knowledge, or psychologically, archetypal content, and are mostly applicable to the community as a whole. These dreams can also be indicative of ancestral displeasure due to the transgression of a spiritual practice or societal taboos and require ceremonies and rituals of appeasement and purification. The two types of dreams are identified as one that corresponds to outer reality and the other that has a deeper, more symbolic meaning.

Once again the remarkable parallel with Jung's conceptualization of dreams is useful here. Jung (1948b) spoke about "insignificant" and "significant" dreams. He explained that

> "little" dreams are the nightly fragments of fantasy coming from the subjective and personal sphere, and their meaning is limited to the affairs of everyday . . . Significant dreams . . . are often remembered for a lifetime, and not infrequently prove to be the richest jewel in the treasure-house of psychic experience. (para. 554)

In a similar fashion to the analyst, the healer approaches the dream with respect for the numinosity of the dream images and messages. The unconscious material, whether communications from the ancestors or psychic manifestations, seems to operate similarly in that the ancestors have a fixed purpose akin to the dream purpose of compensation, correcting an imbalance as well as encapsulating the drive toward wholeness and individuation.

Within the African healing system, as in many other indigenous healing systems, there is an additional valence given to the dream world. In my experience, this valence is at times also present in deep Jungian analysis. For the traditional African healer the dreams carry "a life of their own." Dreams are not only manifestations of the unconscious psyche but are given the status of objective manifestations, with their own ontological reality and consciousness. The dream has an awareness of the dreamer beyond a manifestation of the dreamer's unconscious psyche. This reflects Jung's statement that there is an "unconscious consciousness" (1948f, p. 5, unpublished work). As von Franz (1980a) adds:

> Probably the unconscious has a material aspect, which is why it knows about matter, because it is matter, it is matter which knows itself, as it were. If this were so, then there would be a dim or vague phenomenon of consciousness even in inorganic matter. (p. 37)

The initiate is encouraged to develop an independent relationship with the dream world. This relationship is deemed to be reciprocal and must be accorded the necessary reverence and respect. As such, the dreamer enters into an exchange with the dream world and the ancestral manifestations encountered. In turn the dream world is influenced by the actions of the dreamer/healer.

A phenomenon that is pertinent to the initiate-healer relationship is the healer's ability to enter the dream world of the initiate. The healers describe this phenomenon as "dreaming the dream onward." This could be mistaken as *participation mystique*; however, this would be an erroneous conclusion. The healer's capacity to dream the dream of the initiate is achieved with full conscious awareness. This can rather be understood psychologically as a level of empathic intuition. This concept is crucial to the experience of healing within this indigenous system and further underlies the frequency of synchronistic occurrences in the realm of healing (see chapter 10). In essence, we can understand the fluidity with which the healers enter into the dream world of the initiate or the patient with the amplification of the alchemical *coniunctio*, a union of opposites between healer and patient, or psyche and matter. In the same manner, healers will not ask patients for symptoms of their illness when consulted. Rather, healers rely on communications from dreams and ancestral spirits in order to discern what is out of balance. The accuracy with which they are able to diagnose is remarkable. To my knowledge, this is not common practice in a depth psychology analysis; however, anecdotal evidence exists to indicate that both Jung and von Franz experienced a similar phenomenon (see Whitney, 1986). A healer related her own experiences:

> The dreams will tell you what you need to know. The dreams are how the ancestors tell you about the healing. For instance, a man came to see me about his wife. I saw immediately that he had dreamt that his wife was being swallowed up by flames while lying in her bed. I told him that she was very ill and would soon die. He said no, she is fine, just she is unhappy. I told him she would soon die. He must bring her to me. But he did not. Then two weeks later I saw the man, and he told me his wife had died in a diabetic coma.

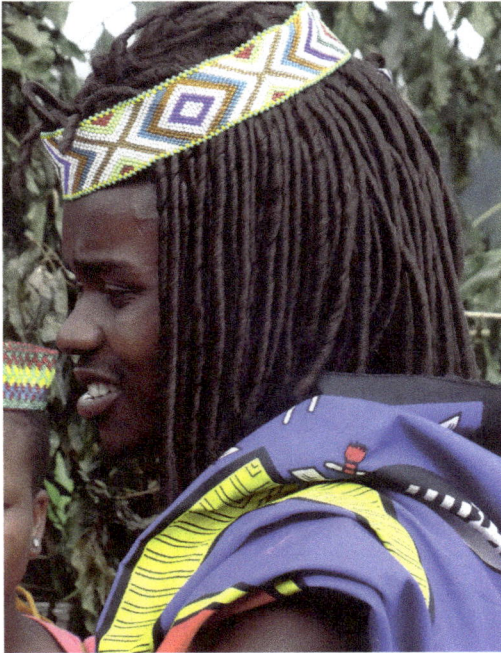

Figure 7. A male healer, Eastern Cape, South Africa

An Initiate's Dream

A dream of an initiate illustrates the approach of the healer to dreams:

I was walking in the forest. I was a young girl in the dream. I had this dress on with an apron, and I was carrying a woven reed basket. The forest was filled with huge trees and in the middle of the forest I found a stone. Then I found a seashell and a bottle filled with sand and a glass marble eye. A figure came to me in the forest and laid his hand on my head. He was immense, tall, and he seemed to glow with light. I knelt down, and he told me I am going to see things differently from other people. The marble was an eye, the all-seeing eye of god, and I will see deeper than others. The stone meant my healing powers and reaching areas that others do not. The shell, because it comes from deep under the waters, was the hidden knowledge and the mysteries that I will learn. The bottle of sands represented was all the people I will help, going all over to bring healing.

This dream was experienced by the initiate as moving and life changing, imbued with numinosity, and it convinced her to follow her calling. The healer's response to the dream would be both concrete and symbolic. On the concrete level, the initiate would be encouraged to actually go and find the objects seen in the dream. These would then become part of her healing tools at a later stage. She would further be encouraged to seek out an actual person who resembles the figure in the dream, who would then become her initiator.

The symbolic understanding of the objects as outlined in the actual dream would be understood to represent the unique qualities of this specific initiate. She would be deemed to have both the healing as well as divining powers as symbolized by the sands, stone, shell, and glass marble eye. Psychologically, we could understand that the dream seems to present a calling for the dreamer to engage with the unconscious and to avail herself of its resources.

The youth of the dreamer indicates that this is the beginning of her journey and that she still has to grow into her gifts and her individuation. She wears an apron, which in the African tradition is associated with the vestments of ritual practice, reminding us of the attire of shamans, signifying levels of stature and occult powers. The apron covers the part of the body that holds the organs of regeneration, fertility, and fecundity (Ronnberg, 2010). It is associated with Adam and Eve and the acquisition of consciousness; Adam and Eve, after eating from the tree of knowledge, sewed fig leaves together and made themselves aprons (Genesis 3:7). The apron of the fire monger or smithy evokes images of the transformative fire. It further symbolizes the feminine, in caring as well as suffocating aspects. To "cut the apron strings" suggests a threshold of maturity and independence.

The dreamer carries a basket, a feminine symbol of containment, often associated with the weaving together of spiritual teachings, a womb-like symbol linked to the mysteries of eternal return, in that it holds corn and seed, symbols of rebirth, regeneration, and fertility. In the dream, the dreamer carries a quaternity of four gifts from the unconscious, found in the unknown and enchanting forest, symbolic of a totality or wholeness.

The forest is the vegetative aspect of the psyche, where unknown dark mysteries reside, often in magical form. Many fairy tales begin in a dark wood, where there is a mysterious quality and where things seem to appear at will and anything is possible. In fairy tales and in the above dream, the forest symbolizes a retreat or a refuge. Von Franz (1982) commented on the meaning of the forest in fairy tales, particularly with respect to the developing feminine. As von Franz noted, venturing in the forest "would mean sinking into one's innermost nature and finding out what it feels like. The vegetative is also spontaneous life and offers healing" (p. 85). It is in the forest that the dreamer, as a young woman, finds a way forward to her own initiation and individuation.

The stone, the shell, the marble eye, and the bottle of sand are all found unexpectedly in the forest. This reminds us that life's gifts are often found in unexpected places. These objects all form part of the divining tools used by some healers for diagnostic purposes. The stone carries the spirit of the ancestor, often marking a place of the gods or place of worship, such as the black stone of Mecca, the Kaaba. It is a symbol of immense qualities, not only suggesting endurance and a sense of eternity, but according to Jung, is *the* symbol of the Self, par excellence. It is the lapis, the philosopher's stone, the symbol of the individual's innermost being and, for the dreamer, a symbol of healing abilities.

The shell evokes images of the great mystery emerging from the unconscious depths, an image of protection, containment, the feminine principle, and Aphrodite's birth (De Vries, 1974). The sand is often combined with the shells and suggests eternity and time passing, like the sands of time. Sand suggests the idea of the multitude and fertility, like the sands on the seashore (Genesis 22:17), the *prima materia* of life as well as movement, change, and transience, symbolized in the image of shifting sands.

The marble eye is yet another of these pregnant symbols of the unconscious psyche. The dream suggests the "all-seeing eye of god," suggesting inner sight, intuition, and eternal knowledge. It will be through her initiation that the neophyte will experience the opening of her eyes to see that which was unknown and to become conscious. The male figure in the dream suggests the great inner man, an ancestral figure or psychopomp, that figure in dreams that guides the soul at times of transition or initiations. He bestows the blessing that launches the dreamer toward a dialogue with the Self. Thus, for the African healer, as it is for the analyst, dreams are the voices of the unknown. In the words of a healer:

Dreams are very important. You have to attend to them immediately. The dreams tell me where to find the herbs and guide me in the process of healing. They are the communications from the ancestors. I know that when I dream of something, a particular thing, it will happen. Your dreams will tell you what you need individually. In one dream, just before the end of my initiation, I was told to go get some leaves from a specific tree and to make *muthi* [healing medicines] from the leaves so that my initiation would go smoothly. When I woke, I went to find the tree. It was exactly where I had seen it in the dream.

Jung (1944) emphasized the importance of the dream symbols in relation to the process of individuation, which is applicable to the initiation system in that he noted these "are images of an archetypal nature which depict the centralizing process or the production of a new centre of the personality" (para. 44). Within the Zulu initiation and healing framework, the presence and the understanding of dreams are necessary precursors to the identification and confirmation of the calling and communications from the ancestors.

Chapter 2
Amadlozi:
The Ancestral Spirits

My body has two lives, my spiritual life and my physical life.
—Ntombi

The journey into the world of African healing, became the discovery that what appears irrational is also rational, both concrete and abstract, symbolic and actual, and portrays the lawfulness of the objective psyche, which contains opposites. Delving into the realms of this cosmology offers us the opportunity to discover the meaning of Jung's (1934a) statement that "psychic reality still exists in its original oneness and awaits man's advance to a level of consciousness where he no longer believes in one part and denies the other, but recognizes both as constituent elements of one psyche" (para. 682). For the African healer, this is embodied in the phenomenon of the ancestors, the living dead.

The ancestral presence represents the subtle spiritual essence of the once-living healer, or family member. Most accounts in the literature, in my experience, do not adequately capture the phenomenon of the ancestors within the African culture. These accounts are often limited by anthropological, sociological, or theological assumptions located predominantly within a Western and/or Christian bias. As such, the idea of the ancestors has been conceived variously as veneration, a cult, idolatrous, or merely as "split-off" aspects of the personality, and projections of an undifferentiated consciousness, all of which are misconstrued. That the ancestors appear as quasi-personal should not be misunderstood as mere projections of human categories or anthropomorphism. Jung (1952b) explained:

All parts of the psyche, inasmuch as they possess a certain autonomy, exhibit a personal character ... But when we go into the matter more deeply, we find that they are really archetypal formations. There are no conclusive arguments against the hypothesis that these archetypal figures are endowed with personality ... and are not just secondary personalizations. In so far as the archetypes do not represent mere functional relationships, they manifest themselves as *daimones*, as personal agencies. In this form they are felt as actual experiences and are not "figments of the imagination," as rationalism would have us believe.... To put it in psychological terms, [man's] consciousness of himself as a personality derives primarily from the influence of quasi-personal archetypes. (para. 388)

The attitude of the healers to the ancestor has further erroneously been interpreted as ancestor worship. This again is the dubious heritage of the missionaries who, while colonizing Africa, vilified the cultural practices that they found, which were different from and independent of Christian doctrines.

Within the African cosmology, the attitude of the living toward the ancestors is one of collaboration, continued remembrance, respect, and affection. The dead—the ancestors—continue to coexist with the living. They continue to cohabit and influence the lives of the living. They participate in daily rituals, and they are given sacred ceremonial positions within the homestead. They are known as the living dead. Jung (1975) observed that "spatial distance is, in the psychic sense, relative," (p. 256) and further, "there are experiences which show that the dead entangle themselves . . . in the physiology of the living" (p. 258).

In the African healing paradigm, "the ancestors form the fulcrum around which the healing epistemology rotates: rituals and ceremonies abound, to appease the ancestors, to learn their wishes, and to be guided by their wisdom" (Radomsky, 2009, p. 36). The seat of the ancestors is always opposite the entrance to the home or in more rural areas, the main entrance to the kraal, or cattle enclosure. Important rituals and ceremonies must be observed when one enters the kraal. It is considered disrespectful to ignore these rituals and to do so risks evoking the wrath of the ancestors.

The communications with the ancestors function to awaken the healer to aspects of the outer life that are out of balance with ancestral needs. These inner stirrings or voices compel the healer to take note and to bring into conscious life the required changes. Serious illness or misfortune is the risk of neglecting these messages. The opposite also applies in that a life lived in accord with the wishes of the ancestors is one in which health and harmony abound. As Jung (1997a) commented, "if one has the right attitude then the right things happen . . . it's as if one is inside of things" (p. 213).

Types of Ancestors

Two groups of ancestors can generally be identified. The first—the *umndiki/mnguni* or *midzimu*—are the blood ancestors, the deceased family members of the individual, and are thus more personal. These ancestors participate in the daily life of individuals and are considered to have human needs, such as the need for warmth, as well as hunger and emotions. They are deemed to be the protective spirits of the living relatives. They often communicate through dreams and visions and mediate between the individual and the spirit world.

The second group of ancestors—known as the *mashovi*—has three sub-types: the first two are *Amadlozi Lomlambo*, the ancestors of the river (see chapter 9) and the *Amadlozi Lehlathi*, the ancestors of the forest. These are recognized as ancestors of other cultures as well as those of nature and of animals. They are not linked to living relatives per se, but are considered to be more universal and more ancient, capable of bestowing certain gifts, such as the ability to heal. They can be understood psychologically as being more numinous and archetypal. The ancestors of this group embody godlike qualities and inspire fear and reverence. These ancestors are exclusive to the healers and are the ancestors of the *ukuthwasa* phase of initiation (see chapter 4). The third subtype includes the *Amadlozi Lengozi*, the angry or vengeful spirits, which are deemed to be malevolent and responsible for evil acts.

The Healer's Relationship to the Ancestors

Within the African cosmology, coincidence does not exist. The primary aim of the ancestors is to encourage a life lived in accord with their wishes, understood psychologically as living in accord with the unconscious. Health, both physical and spiritual, is a direct result of such an accord. Illness or misfortune is a disturbance in the relationship with the ancestors.

The healer is said to have access to understanding the will of the ancestors and is thus capable of mediating between the ancestral spirits and the living. The healers thus embody the seat of cultural knowledge and traditional mythology, simultaneously a part of the individual's reality as well as the greater communal whole and ancestral realm. A healer explains the relationship between the ancestors and the individual:

> I believe what I am made of, this body, is an arrangement between two sides: the physical and the spiritual. When I die, that spiritual part, the soul, that part still communicates even though the body is no longer living. These are the ancestors, and they communicate with God. We see the signs of their existence in dreams; it is as if your mind suddenly comes alive and tells you where to find things, gives solutions to your problems, your healing. You could not just be that wise, you are not that brilliant just to know these things. It is the ancestors showing you the way.

Another healer describes the ancestral connection this way:

> There are two souls *Ena* and *Moya*. Moya is the great soul part of the person, connected to God. There is a good and evil part to Moya. Each needs to be in balance with the other. If there is an imbalance, the person gets ill. Ena is more closely linked with the person and "looks" like the person. This is the part that grows with the person as the person lives his life depending on his experiences.

These two souls are also described as one being vegetative, which dies with the body, and the other being spiritual, which lives on and that has an effect on the living as well as a consciousness that survives death. Again Jung's (1977) reflections are helpful psychologically in that he said, "few people know anything about the ancestral soul and even fewer believe in it. Why is it so difficult to believe that each of us has two souls?" (p. 57).

The healers link their worldview to their own ancestors and to the ancestors of their patients. Healer, patient, and ancestors form the system of relationships that molds the treatment procedures. A similar relationship develops between the healer and the initiate during an initiation process.

I have come to understand, psychologically, the healer's relationship to the ancestors as being perhaps symbolic of the ego-Self axis, that living vein of psychic dialogue between consciousness and the unconscious or autonomous numinous psychic content. Through the initiation process, the healer is able to withstand the demands of the ancestors without being overwhelmed or succumbing to a psychosis or inflation. By respecting the call from the ancestors, the ego is placed in a living relationship to the Self. As von Franz (1998) observed: "The effect of archetypal motifs can be blinding or it can be culturally constructive; it can lead to the . . . highest spiritual creations [which depends on] whether the individual is able to preserve his ego-consciousness" (p. 137).

The communications between the ancestors and the healer is an active dialogue that can be compared to Jung's process of active imagination, in which there are both conscious viewpoints and autonomous expressions of the unconscious psyche. Jung (1977) described this relationship thus:

> Supposing the spirit has a subjective existence, a consciousness of its own, then there also exists an ethical relation to what it is or what it wants or what it needs. And if I live in such a way that it helps this spirit, it is a moral achievement. (p. 385)

The understanding of the relationship to the ancestors is complex and challenging. Jung (1957a) observed that "we fear and reject with horror any sign of living sympathy, partly because a sympathetic understanding might permit contact with an alien spirit to become a serious experience" (para. 1).

For the African healer, this phenomenon is connected to three broad concepts, those of kinship, death, and relationship to the land. There is an African proverb that says: "One tree cannot make a forest. For a forest to develop all the individual trees must lend their roots and their branches." This is also captured in the saying "*Umuntu ngumuntu ngabantu*," a phrase that colloquially has become known as *Ubuntu*, or "I am because you are." This concept of kinship and continued coexistence is not severed in death.

The Western view of death is often mostly spatial. That is, in death there is a permanent removal of the deceased person, the concept of

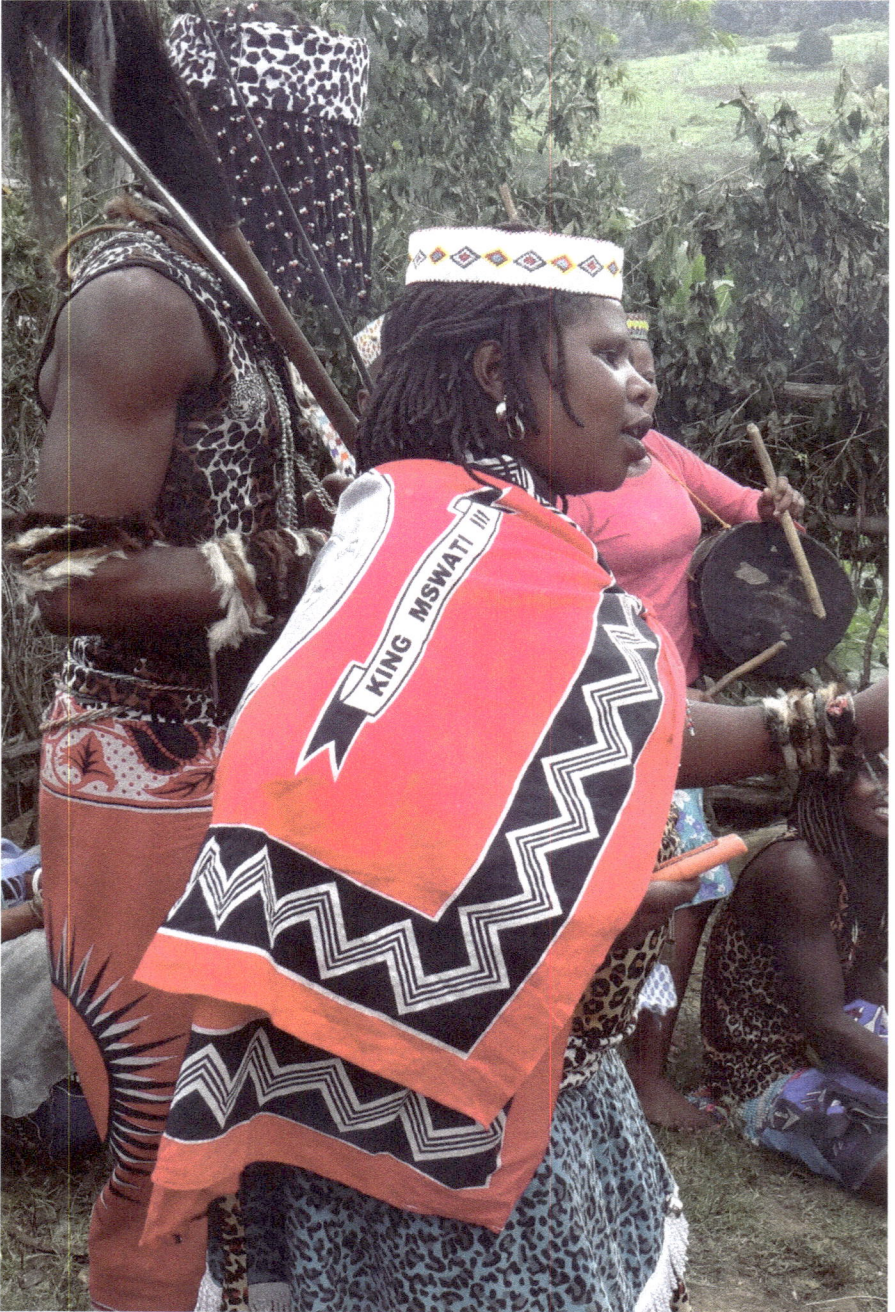

Figure 8. A healer dressed in the traditional regalia known as *amabhayi*

finality, a termination of life, where the dead are spoken of in the past tense. In the African system, death is understood in terms of kinship. The dead have a continued presence, and death is considered a change in status rather than a termination. In other words, death does not extinguish kinship ties. Jung (1977) reflected on the idea of consciousness after death, and he said:

> At least parts of our psyche are not subject to the laws of space and time, otherwise perceptions outside of space and time would be impossible—yet they exist. Our conceptions of space and time as seen from the causal rationalistic standpoint are incomplete. (p. 377)

And further:

> I am convinced that if the European had to go through the same exercises and ceremonies which the medicine man performs in order to make spirits visible, he would have the same experiences. He would . . . of course, devalue them. (1948d, para. 573)

Life, Death, and the Afterlife

The theme of life, death, and the afterlife is one that permeates this work, weaving the web that embeds the phenomenon of the ancestors within the African healing paradigm. The African healer exists on a day-to-day basis in that liminal space between the living and the dead, or between the consciousness and the unconscious, between psyche and matter. For the healer, this threshold, which Western science has largely dismissed, is a natural and necessary part of life. The dichotomy and dislocation between life and death is foreign to the epistemology of the healer. I do not mean to suggest that the healer only exists in a state of undifferentiated uroboric regressive unconsciousness, but rather, that the healer with conscious awareness traverses this domain, holding both sides in a respectful union.

In her seminal work, *On Dreams and Death* (1987), von Franz posed pertinent questions that underscore this material, such as: Does survival after death, if it exists, continue only for a time or for longer? How do the dead relate to each other or to the living? Does the personality of the deceased disintegrate after death? And so forth. Over time, I have put some of these questions to various healers. What always astounds me, no matter how often I hear it or experience it, is the lack of uncertainty with which these questions are answered. Mostly I'm met with an indulgent bemusement and patience for this ignorant Western person who is asking such obvious things.

Von Franz (1986) commented on the importance of the motifs in the dreams of the dying in that "we may have before us what are obviously the most natural psychic images of the death process and life after death" (p. xiii). On reflection, I would ask whether the dreams and ancestral communications of the healers offer us a unique *living* model of the same. What is of interest in comparison to the work of von Franz are the similarities of the motifs in the dreams of the healers, the themes of death and resurrection, and transformation into the living dead, or the ancestors.

The symbols that appear in death dreams echo those that manifest in the individuation process, as von Franz (1986) stated unequivocally: "In principle, individuation dreams do not differ in their archetypal symbolism from death dreams" (p. xiii). I venture to add: nor do they differ from the dreams of the healers during and after the initiation process. These archetypal themes circumambulate over and over whether we are talking about individuation, death, resurrection, or initiation. These themes include: separation and dismemberment, a great passage or journey, the crossing of a threshold, the presence of companions, the completion of tasks, the transformation of the physical into the spiritual, a return, and a rebirth or resurrection.

A further differentiation is also noted by von Franz (1986) between when the figure of a dead person in a dream is being used as a symbol for the dreamer's inner reality and when the figure represents an actual deceased person. This differentiation between the subjective and the objective interpretation is one that is often not immediately apparent when it comes to the phenomenon of the ancestors.

Psychologically, this relationship between the healer and ancestors can be understood perhaps as the ego having a respectful and authentic attitude toward the manifestations of the autonomous psyche, in that each is aware of the other and both are influenced by the other. The healer lives in accord with the ancestors, observes the communications from the ancestors, caters to their needs, and thus receives something back that is transformative, while the ancestors in turn are shaped by the healer's interactions.

Recent developments in modern science, especially in quantum physics and quantum mechanics, seem to be slowly creeping toward the borders of that hinterland that the indigenous healers—and Jung and von Franz—were able to intuit and experience. This includes the phenomena of non-locality and of entanglement: the fact that subatomic particles can exist in two places simultaneously and that light behaves both as a wave and a particle. What seems to be required is a move toward what the healers, ancient alchemists, and mystics know: The unity of psyche and matter and the presence of spirit in nature.

To be clear, what I am hoping to uncover through this journey into the realm of the African healer is the idea of the level of reality underlying the unconscious psyche expressed in the form of trans-psychic phenomenon specific to the realm of the healers and the phenomenon of the ancestors. This journey further offers a glimpse of what Jung called the *psychoid*, an unconscious behind which something unknowable and trans-psychic is at work, and the unexpected parallelism of psychic and physical events. The psychoid nature is such that what appears in one instance as a psychic image also appears as a physical event (see chapter 10). Von Franz (1992) explained that the term *psychoid* denotes "the fact that the archetypes of the objective psyche sometimes . . . cross over into the realm of matter. . . . This seems to confirm . . . the possibility of a *unus mundus* and an ultimate unity of physical and psychic energy" (p. 251).

This differs from the idea of ancestors conceptualized as unconscious complexes related to our personal histories.

Jung (1948d) initially considered these phenomena as projections of the personal complex when he wrote "parapsychic phenomena . . . are . . . the exteriorized effects of unconscious complexes . . . and I must regard this whole territory as an appendix to psychology" (para. 600). He later revised this assertion when he reflected:

> After collecting psychological evidence from many people and many countries for fifty years, I no longer feel as certain as I did in 1919 . . . To put it bluntly, I doubt whether an exclusively psychological approach can do justice to the phenomenon in question . . . Findings on parapsychology as well as the realm of nuclear physics and the conception of the space-time continuum

. . . opens up the whole question of the trans-psychic reality immediately underlying the psyche. (1948d, para. 600, n. 15)

When considering these phenomena, Jung was naturally ambivalent, at times confirming and other times disconfirming his thoughts on this issue, perhaps restrained by the zeitgeist of his day. Jung resolved this conflict by focusing exclusively on the psychological aspect of this phenomenon. He said:

I have confined myself . . . to the psychological side of the problem . . . as . . . it is extraordinarily difficult to find reliable evidence for the independent existence of spirits . . . since (these) are as a rule nothing but very ordinary products of the personal unconscious . . . *There are nevertheless, a few exceptions.* (1948d, para. 599; emphasis added)

The phenomena of the living dead seem to be one of the exceptions referred to by Jung while also offering the opportunity to explore the trans-psychic realm underlying the psyche. Jung (1948e) commented, "though our critical arguments may cast doubt . . . there is not a single argument that could prove that spirits do not exist" (para. 748). Still today, one hesitates to speak too candidly about such phenomena, and I do wonder how Jung would have responded to contact with the healers and the realm of the *amadlozi*.

The African healing system cannot be differentiated into neat secular versus sacred categories; rather the sense of the sacred permeates all life all the time. The relationship to the ancestors is a way of seeing and understanding the world and is not a religious system, although a religious attitude is required. Jung (1948d) was aware of this, and he commented in reference to an indigenous person that

his belief in spirits, or rather, his awareness of the spiritual world, pulls him again and again out of that bondage in which his senses hold him; it forces on him the certainty of a spiritual reality whose laws he must observe as carefully and as guardedly as the laws of his physical environment. . . . Physical reality is at the same time spiritual reality. (para. 572)

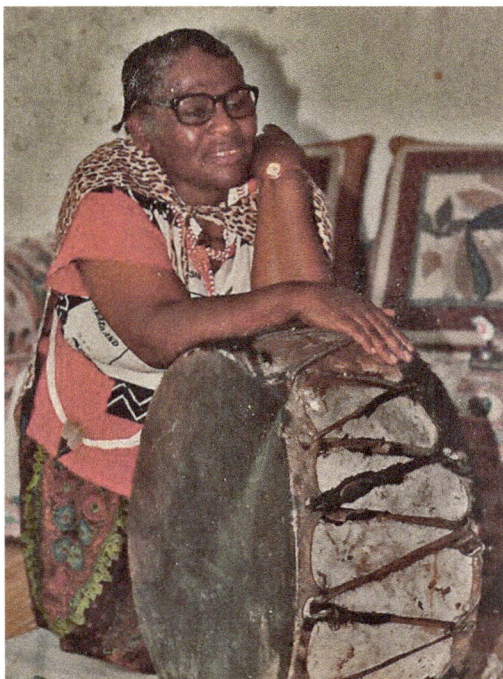

Figure 9. Healer with a cowhide drum

Parapsychological and synchronistic phenomena belong here, too (see chapter 10 for further discussion). For the healer, these events belong to an objective reality of the ancestral spirit having an impact on material reality. Psychologically, we continue to hold the question of whether these events are in fact a window opening between two realms, a *fenestra eternis,* or products of the unconscious complexes of the individual involved or activated contents of the collective unconscious. As von Franz (1974) observed, these "are parapsychological phenomena . . . prone to take place in the life of an individual when a gradient of energy exists between the conscious and unconscious . . . when archetypal content is in an excited state" (p. 246).

It is my view and experience that all of the above are valid at different times and in different contexts, but that none can be reduced to a *nothing-but* experience. We know, thanks to Jung, that there is what he called "absolute knowledge" in the unconscious (1948d, para. 572). Here Jung postulates an *a priori* meaning in nature. The unconscious knows what we do not yet know consciously. Within the African healing culture, this relationship to unconscious knowledge is captured in the relationship of the living to the living dead and is forged through the initiation ceremonies.

As I sat writing these words, questions came to me: Would the ancestors approve of what I am doing? Can I speak of these things? Have I been mindful enough of acting in accord with the unconscious? At that very moment when these questions were plaguing my thoughts and I found myself unable to continue writing, a cowhide drum, which sits in the corner of my writing room, emitted a loud explosive sound. As the drum is one used during a number of ceremonies to symbolize the ancestors voicing their approval (see chapter 3), perhaps, the cowhide drum emitting an explosive sound at that particular moment when I was seeking some reassurance may have had a similar meaning. In the very least, it was a synchronistic event, which generally signifies that the archetypal energies are stirring.

Chapter 3
Ukuphahla:
Connecting with Spirit

This is how I answered the ancestral way.
The way to becoming the healer.
—Ntombi

Ntombi had arrived at the beginning of her analysis in a state of agitation and exhaustion. She had lost interest in her life, her studies, and her relationship. She had become increasingly withdrawn and isolated. Her presentation reflected the state of confusion and dis-union, which the alchemists referred to as the *massa confusa*, the primordial state that is experienced as a darkness and loss of direction, but also often holds the seeds of transformation. Ntombi related a dream, which seemed to compensate for her conscious state of mind and to hint at the way forward:

Two men and a woman approach me. The leader is the tallest, strong and muscular. He is dressed in plain clothes, but he is adorned with the beads of a healer. He is very stern and he insists that I go with him.

This dream was followed by a synchronistic encounter with a healer. Ntombi met a woman in a shop who approached her and identified herself as an initiate. She invited Ntombi to accompany her to witness her inauguration ritual as a novice healer. Ntombi expressed a deep fear at the idea of attending the ceremony. As we explored her anxieties, she reflected:

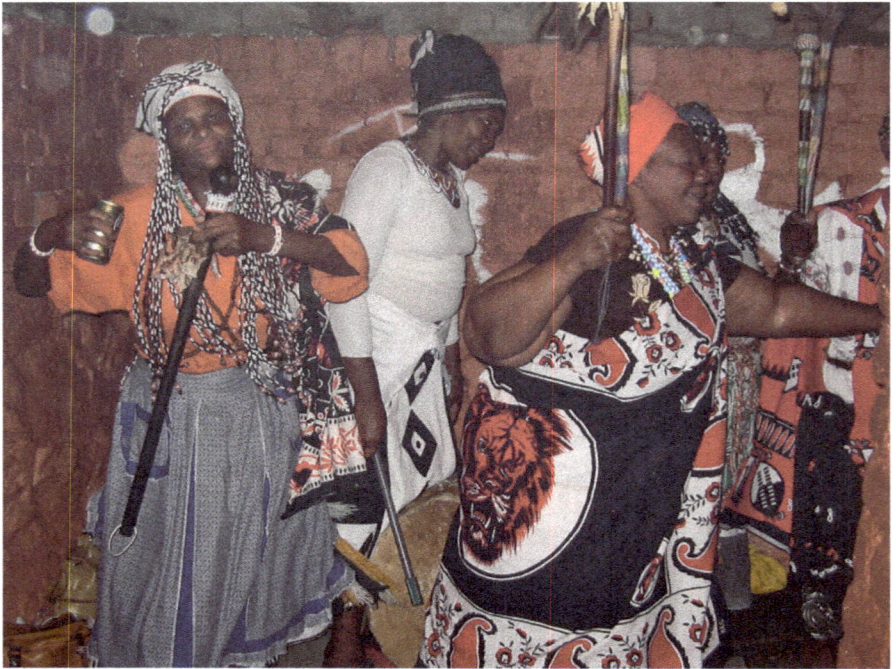

Figure 10. Healers participate in an initiation dance ceremony

I know if I go to this ceremony, then I will no longer be able to deny the calling. It keeps happening you see, wherever I go, in the streets, in the shops, healers stop me and tell me that they can "see" that I need to undergo the initiation. The dreams too, I know that I need to accept this, but it terrifies me. What about my life?

The most obvious and concrete encounter with the practice of African healing is in the form of the dance, song, and drumming rituals. These ceremonies abound in different forms throughout the initiation process. When one observes and participates in the various rituals it becomes clear that the function of the ritual action is to impose a certain form on instinctual or archetypal energies. In so doing, a transformation of libido to higher form of consciousness occurs. The resultant outcome of the repetitive ritualized actions, in which high levels of libido are accessed, is the overcoming of ego constraints and an opening up to the transpersonal. Psychologically, these rituals aim toward the development of consciousness in the initiate, from a *participation mystique* toward a more differentiated consciousness that ultimately facilitates a connection to the Self.

Jung (1954c) commented that with ritual action "man places himself at the disposal of an autonomous and eternal agency operating outside the categories of human consciousness" (para. 379). Neumann (1954) explained that this means that the ego complex has the capacity to submerge into the unconscious, while retaining a kernel of consciousness, gain experience and knowledge, remember and return with the boon (p. 330).

In the African healing paradigm, this "autonomous and eternal agency" takes the form of the phenomenon of the ancestors. In this realm, the transpersonal numinosum is experienced in the form of trance, which is a well-known shamanic experience but difficult to explain. During the trance, the ego submits temporarily to the unconscious, allowing the transpersonal to predominate. The healer moves at will in and out of the transpersonal matrix, while retaining full recall of this experience. In this realm, the transpersonal experience can thus become a personal one. Jung (1940) was aware of the power of the sacred, the numinous, as that "invisible presence that causes a peculiar alteration of consciousness." (para.6) In essence, psychologically, this means that through the dance, the repetition of ritual movements, and the song, clapping, and drumming, the libido is diverted and in the service of the unconscious.

Jung (1948a) noted that through the meaning of the ritual the transpersonal numinosum is experienced (para.104). Here, in the realm of ancestral knowledge, the purely personal is transcended and something transpersonal emerges. The initiation ritual further aims to develop ego strength in order to facilitate the encounter with the unconscious and to guard against becoming possessed by or identified with autonomous unconscious forces.

The Healing Dance Ceremony

A central aspect of the healing and initiation process is the *intlombe*, a specific form of ceremonial dance.[10] The complexity and nature of the ceremony varies according to different healing or initiation needs. The aim of the ceremony is the awakening of ancestral energies into their full numinosity. These rituals function psychologically to help the participant

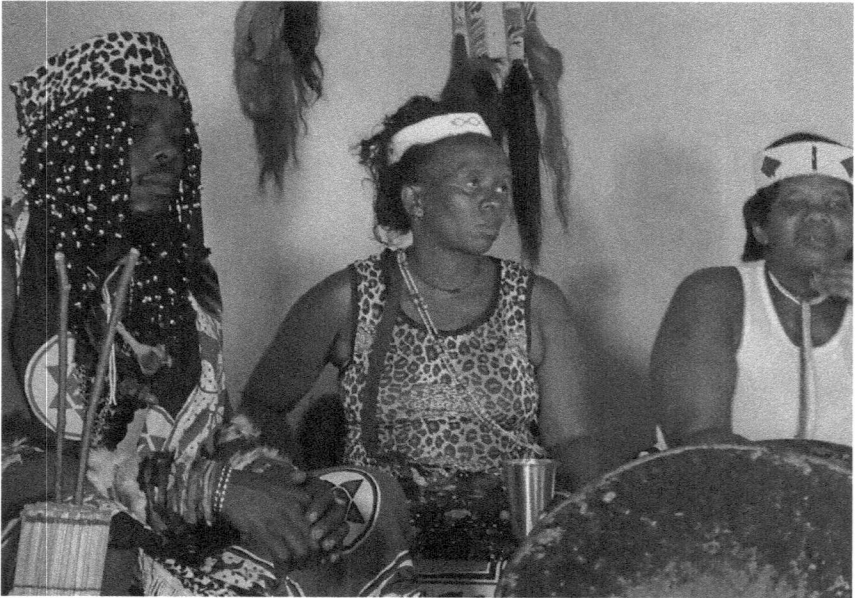

Figure 11. Healers participate in ritual *intlombe* ceremony inside the hut

detach from a preceding stage of development and transfer psychic energy to the next stage.

The ceremonies are always performed inside the healer's hut or enclosure, and the basic ritual structure is always the same. In rural areas where the authentic rituals take place, the huts are round with a reed roof. The round walls of the healer's hut form the temenos or the retort that contains the numinous energies evoked in the ritual. The drummer sits against the wall of the hut facing the doorway, in the place of the ancestors.

Inside the hut, family and community members form a circle, men on the right-hand side of the entrance and women to the left of the doorway. These people participate and support the ritual by singing and clapping with the drumbeat. Inside this circle, the healers and initiates dance in a counterclockwise circular direction as the aim of this dance is a rejuvenation. The center of the hut is marked by a raised fireplace or a central pole. Bare feet pound the clay earthen ground in time with the drums, the ceremonial songs, and the clapping. The dance continues in a repetitive circular rhythm, circumambulating the central core of the hut in order to induce heavy sweating and to raise the *moya* or spirit.

This circular movement evokes the alchemical operation of *circulatio*, the repeated movement up and down, or round and round in order for something to change. This repetitive circular movement is often present in the analytical process. Complexes and old attitudes are revisited time and again, mirroring this circular movement, before a new realization dawns or something transforms. Edinger (1991) explains:

> Psychologically, *circulatio* is the repeated circuit of all aspects of one's being, which gradually generates awareness of a transpersonal centre uniting the conflicting factors. There is a transit through the opposites, which are experienced alternatively again and again, leading finally to their reconciliation. (pg. 143)

As a healer reflected, "the dancing is to help to move the energy of the ancestors and to help you to speak to them." This continues for long periods, often all night, with the resultant release of endorphins and induction of a trance.

The dance ritual is permeated with an atmosphere of physical and psychological vitality. Jung (1952b) observed the dance rhythms of the Pueblo and reflected that it is the bare feet themselves as well as the hard pounding of the earth that symbolize fertility, in that the purposeful rhythm activates, organizes, and channels the libido into a new form of activity downward toward Mother Earth. As Jung (1952b) explained:

> The regression of the libido makes the ritual act of treading out the dance step seem like a repetition of the infantile "kicking" . . . and recapitulates a movement that was already practiced in the mother's womb. The foot and the treading movement are invested with a phallic significance . . . so that the rhythm of the dance transports the dancer into an unconscious state. (para. 481)

For the healers, the dance is the elixir that initiates the trance, accompanied by a personal song. Each initiate is said to "hear" their song in the trance. This song becomes the healing song as well as a validation of the authenticity of the calling. The songs are a symbolic narrative of ancestral experiences. A healer shared his dream in which his song was revealed to him:

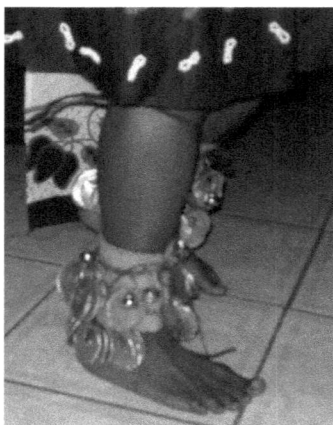

Figure 12. *Amafahlawana*: ankle bracelets worn during the dance ceremony

I attend a gathering. My family is there as well. I'm standing alone to one side. I sense that I am there for some purpose, but I'm not sure what. In the center of the gathering is a clearing. In the middle of the clearing a group of healers are dancing and singing. I look down at my feet and in a bag on the ground are all the garments I will need for my regalia. I slowly start to dress in the regalia. Then I notice that the healers are waiting for me to join them in the center of the circle. We dance and one healer tells me to listen for my song. I know that my song will come. I wake with a sense of peace and my song in my mind.

The dance ritual is punctuated by the healers performing *vumisa*, an altered state of consciousness in which they communicate with the ancestors and evoke healing. C.A. Meier (1989) noted that dancing and music has "a particularly rousing effect, producing enthusiasm in which the soul becomes capable of soothsaying" (p. 87). The enthusiasm is palpable at this time and reflects the original meaning of the word—*enthous*, or inspired by God. Questions are addressed to the healers, who convey information to the ancestors, the healers acting as the intermediaries. The healers describe this as "listening and hearing with ears of mystery." The participants in these dance rituals describe feelings of vitality, both physical and spiritual.

Von Franz (1980b) explained that the mobilization of physical energy through the activation of psychic energy in the dance and drumming rhythms transforms physiological aspects into spiritual forms. The activation of the spiritual energy opens the pathway to the transpersonal, or the Self. As von Franz (1997b) noted:

> The Self is not static . . . it is more often represented by some moving or dancing body . . . The secret is to be able to follow it, to dance with it, because the Self is constantly performing a dance, a circular movement of eternal renewal. (p. 65)

The archetype of the dance is rich and diverse. To note just a few amplifications: Shiva Nataraja, Lord of Dance, awakens matter through dance; Jesus performs a mystical dance with the apostles while his body is crucified in the apocryphal acts of St. John; David danced before the "Lord with all his might" (Chronicle 15:29; Samuel 6:14). Dance is pivotal in Islamic mysticism and the Dervish orders, where the dance is seen as a direct portal to divine influence. Wosien (1974) observed that "in whatever form dance presents itself, it always aims at approaching the god . . . As an act of sacrifice, as man giving himself to his god, the dance is total surrender" (p. 9).

The purpose of the ritual dance of the African healer seems to be to strive for wholeness, for contact with that which is beyond duality, and to be in touch with the *unus mundus*. A healer described her understanding of the central role of dance in the rituals:

> The dance is very important. Here we use the drums and dance around and around in a circle. It is a praise dance for the ancestors, but it also calls the energy to help heal or to solve a problem. There is a lot of energy, and the healers will sometimes fall into a trance during the dance, and the ancestors will speak through them. We welcome the ancestors and listen to their guidance. It is a way to raise the energy and to clear the mind and the body to be open to the ancestors.

Jung (1954c) observed:

> The aim and the effect of the . . . round dance is to impress upon the mind the image of the circle and the center and the relation of each point along the periphery to that center. Psychologically, this arrangement is equivalent to a mandala and is thus a symbol of the self. (para. 419)

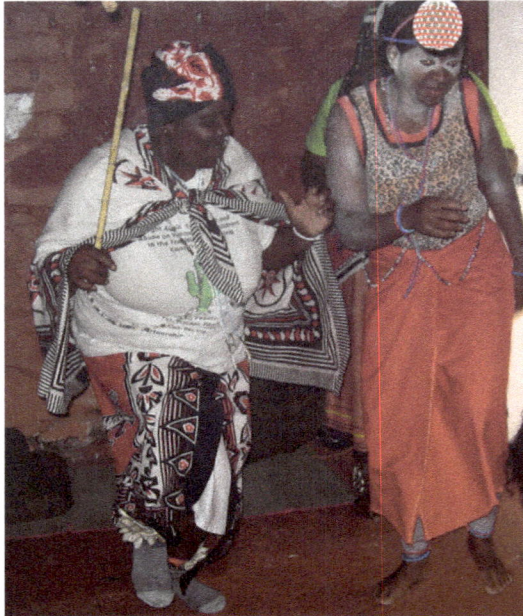

Figure 13. Healers dance during the *intlombe*

The Living Mandala

An aerial view of this ceremony reveals a living, dancing mandala. These dances and songs are never arbitrary, and the movements follow an unspoken intuitive pattern. The mandala formation, according to Jung (1944, para. 174), is an archetypal form that functions to concentrate libido toward one central point. This potentially unites disintegrative forces such as opposites, permitting a regeneration and rebirth of new attitudes or new consciousness. These ceremonies as a whole seem reflective of Neumann's (1955) observations that: "originally all ritual was dance in which the whole corporeal psyche was literally set into motion" (p. 295), or in Jung's (1944) words:

> The rites are attempts to abolish the separation between the conscious mind and the unconscious, the real source of life, and to bring about a reunion of the individual with the native soil of his inherited, instinctive make-up. (para. 174)

The symbol of the mandala has the meaning of a holy place, a temenos, a means of protecting the center of the personality from being drawn out and influenced by outer distractions. As Jung (1955–56) explained, "the mandala symbolizes, by it' central point, the ultimate unity of all archetypes as well as the multiplicity of the phenomenal world, and is therefore the empirical equivalent of the metaphysical concept of a *unus mundus*" (para. 661). Thus, in turn, it represents an ultimate oneness of inner and outer reality. The effect of the mandala and how it reacts upon its maker is described by Jung (1962):

> Very ancient magical effects lie hidden in this symbol for it derives originally from the "enclosing circle," the "charmed circle," the magic of which has been preserved in countless folk customs. The image has the obvious purpose of drawing a *sulcus primigenius*, a magical furrow around the center, the *templum* or *temenos* (sacred precinct), of the innermost personality in order to prevent "flowing out," or to guard by apotropaic means against deflections through external influences. . . . That is to say, by means of these concrete performances, the attention . . . or the interest, is brought back to an inner sacred domain, which is the source and the goal of the soul and which contains the unity of life and consciousness. The unity once possessed has been lost, and must now be found again. (pp. 102–103)

In the dance, this effect is immediately apparent, and the idea emerges that rhythmic sound in cosmogenic myths is at the root of all creation. Wosien (1974) observed "through the ritualized dance of the healer, one comes into contact with the archaic layers of the self, the realm of the gods, who are alive and well" (p. 7).

In my experience, all who attend, observe, or participate in such a ceremony come away with a sense of awe, an indescribable sensation that the healers explained as "something you cannot put into words, but only feel in your body." Thus the effect of these rituals seems to be that of connecting the realm of the archetypes with the outer phenomenal world. This ritualized physical embodiment of the symbolic meaning of the mandala is lacking in the more static activity of drawing a mandala. The transformative effect of the physical activity is immense and facilitates the downgrading of the ego position thus making room for the emergence of the unconscious, the psychical, and the spiritual. To me, it seems that the moving mandala puts the dancer in direct contact with the organizing principle of the Self. A dream of an initiate reflects this archetypal image:

> *I have been given a task that will be part of my final preparations. As part of my preparations I have to learn a certain dance that can only be learnt in the bowels of an ancient tree. Inside the tree is a large clearing and on the ground is a multicolored circular design embedded in the clearing. Here I will learn to dance.*

The Voice of the Drums

Central to the dance is the steady rhythm of the drum. The drum is one of the most ancient of musical instruments and has been used throughout antiquity and mythology to induce trance states for healing and prophesying. The drum and the drumming form a central part of all healing rituals. The drumbeat reflects the pulse of life, the heartbeat. This in turn evokes the elemental powers, activating the processes of creation and linking the individual to the rhythms of the cosmos. The round edge of the drum is said to mirror that horizon beyond which the healer journeys, carrying the healer into altered states of consciousness and also calling the healer back to consciousness, an anchor in matter (Ronnberg, 2010).

The drum is seen as the call to activity, the voice that awakens the ancestors and focuses their attention on the ritual and the need for healing guidance. The drummers' central position within the hut facing the entrance way, the seat of the ancestors, is deliberate, and ceremonies cannot be successful without this aspect.

The healing aspect and the voice of the drum are known as *ngoma* (Radomsky & Levers, 2012). The *sangoma* is the healer who performs the ritual. Embedded within the meanings of the name is the realization that the healer is a vehicle for the voice of the ancestors.

The drums of the healers are characteristically made from the skins of the sacrificial animals that participated in the healer's own initiation process. The healers explain that the animal spirit of the hide was thought to return with the beating of its skin. Thus the spirit of the animal resides in the skin

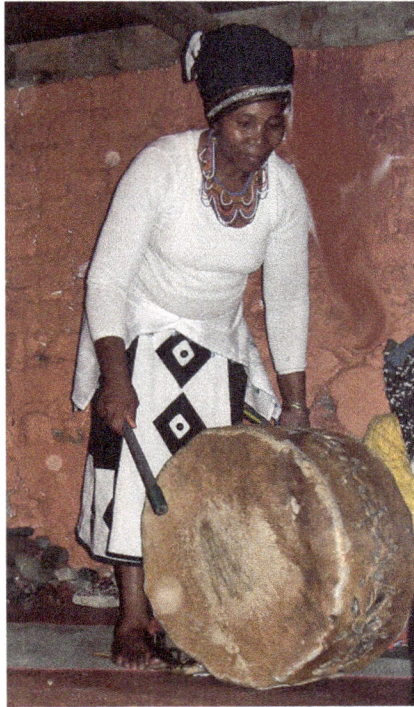

Figure 14. A *sangoma* drumming at a healing ritual

and evokes an image of spirit in matter. Jung (1939) summed up the essence of the ritual as follows:

> Man expresses his most fundamental and most important psychological conditions in ritual . . . the ritual is the cult performance of these basic psychological facts. That explains why we should not change anything in a ritual. A ritual must be done according to tradition . . . in former centuries man did not need that kind of intellectual understanding . . . We are not far enough advanced psychologically to understand . . . the extraordinary truth of ritual. (para. 617)

The voice of the drum and the movement of the dance form the temenos for the transformational effect of the initiation ritual central to the calling.

Chapter 4
Ukuthwasa:
A Call to Healing

I alone had to carry on the true family way and become a healer.
That was my burden in life.
—Ntombi

Ntombi's awareness of the burden of her calling was expressed in her evocative and distressing plea: "Please make the dreams go away." She had suffered an *abaissement du niveau mental*, a kind of lowering of consciousness and loss of soul. Jung (1946b, para. 477) suggested that in such a state there is the experience of a loss of initiative where the conscious mind is in danger of surrendering to the power of the unconscious. At the outset her condition seemed to embody the zeitgeist of contemporary South Africa. On a collective level, she was a black woman struggling to emerge from a segregationist and racialist past within a society still bound by prejudicial and intolerant autocratic values. On a personal level, she was facing the upsurge of terrifying autonomous psychic forces.

It was clear that the demands of the calling and all that would be required of her psychologically fuelled her conflict. Ntombi's fear of and resistance to her calling was a fear of the irrational and of the eruptions from the autonomous psyche. Jung (1961a) commented that "whenever there is a reaching down into innermost experience . . . most people are overcome with fright . . . the possibility that such experience might have psychic reality is anathema to them" (p. 164). Ultimately, psychologically, her fear could be understood as a fear of God, the numinous or the Self. I was reminded of Jung's words when he said, "God is the name by which I designate all things that cross my willful path violently and recklessly, all things which upset my subjective views, plans and intentions and change the course of my life for better or worse" (in Edinger, 1972, p. 101). Yet behind the fear, as became apparent in the work with Ntombi, lay something teleological, which could pave the way to individuation.

Ntombi's rational view of her life was positive in that she had achieved much under difficult circumstances. However, she then came face-to-face with an ethical conflict, which she experienced as a call from something that was anathema to her, from all that had been rejected by her family's acculturation. She was being called to be true to her inner nature. She was faced with honoring this or remaining steadfast in the artificial collective life she had adopted. Her fear was centered on the realization of self-sacrifice that would be required in order to live a more authentic life. Jung (1953) reminds us that this fear "lurks deep in every ego . . . Fear that is often only the attempt to precariously control the demands of the unconscious forces . . . No one who strives for individuation is spared this dangerous passage" (para. 849).

Ntombi would face a number of challenges as her fear was also embedded in her personal life history: Her grandfather had faced the task imposed on him by the unconscious and had taken up the mantle of the healer. But her father had rejected his culture and adopted a God-image that did not hold for her. As Ntombi reflected:

> That is why my illness was so bad. I was, so to say, "ill" for the whole family. For the generations that could not recognize their calling. My father had the church, the Christian church, but he was unhappy all the time. I believe that he had lost his roots. He was not who he should have been and therefore he could never be happy.

Ntombi too had tried to escape her roots. She had escaped into a scientific and rational one-sidedness, and she had forsaken the mystery of her culture. In this she no longer lived a symbolic life but rather lived in contradiction to her nature. Thus her fear was also the fear of the unrealized inner God-image, an unrealized aspect of the Self. The very thing that she most feared would prove to be her salvation. The calling, paradoxically, would provide Ntombi with a way to approach and assimilate her fear.

Jung (1931) noted the "alienation from the unconscious and from its historical conditions spells rootlessness . . . for every individual who through a one-sided allegiance to any kind of -ism, loses touch with the dark material earthy ground of his being" (para. 103). While the process of becoming a Western-trained biomedical doctor was, for Ntombi, one predominantly of conscious choice, the calling to become a healer is a call from the unconscious.

The Calling as a Creative Process

The evolution of the African healer is not a personal conscious choice but rather a calling. This process is known colloquially in the Zulu tradition as *ukuthwasa. Ukuthwasa* is the initiatory illness and the necessary preliminary stage that drives the sufferer to accept the calling of becoming a healer. *Ukuthwasa* refers to "the beginning" or "the emergence of something new" and implies that a transformation will take place in the person in the acceptance of the calling. From the African healing perspective, once the calling is recognized, there is no choice but to follow its path.

The term *ukuthwasa* is both a noun and a verb. It is a term that describes the preliminary illness that identifies the calling as well as the initiation of the Zulu healing process. The aim is to bring to the fore new aspects or potentials in the individual that have remained dormant or unconscious. Once the calling is identified and accepted by the initiate and the healer, the initiate is said to *thwasa* and is colloquially referred to as a *thwasa*, literally, "the one undergoing the *ukuthwasa* initiation."

To be chosen is the central theme of the individuation process where the ego encounters the Self. One is given a task with personal and trans-personal purpose, singled out and required to pay constant attention to inner stirrings. Marie-Louise von Franz commented that the process of individuation or "the conscious coming-to-terms with one's own inner center . . . or Self—generally begins with a wounding of the personality and the suffering that accompanies it. This initial shock amounts to a sort of a 'call'" (quoted in Jung 1990, p. 166).

Psychologically, the call is an archetypal experience that potentially initiates individuation and births the awareness of a transpersonal other. As such, the calling can be understood as a threshold phenomenon that initiates a creative process. As will become clear, the initiate in an original state of a pre-conscious, undifferentiated wholeness suffers a shift in energy that is initially experienced as a state of disillusionment. Jung (1973, p. 496) spoke of the energy gradient between consciousness and the unconscious. He explained that in order for a creative process to unfold, there needs to be a lowering of the energy gradient at the threshold of consciousness. With this shift in the energy gradient, unconscious content breaks into consciousness, disrupting the original unity and resulting in a shift in consciousness. The *ukuthwasa* initiation functions to develop sufficient ego strength in order for the initiate to withstand the change in the energy gradient and the resultant upsurge of unconscious energy without falling into an inflation or psychosis.

The signs of the *ukuthwasa* illness include both physical and psychological symptoms that do not respond to medical treatment and are often debilitating for the sufferer. Many initiates report symptoms diagnosed as serious illnesses. Most sufferers consult Western medical doctors but in many cases without success. Some of the initiates report invasive and painful treatments or operations in the attempt to confirm a medical diagnosis. Other initiates report symptoms that mimic psychopathological illnesses such as major depression, psychosis, and schizophrenia. Many, out of ignorance or fear, end up in treatment programs in psychiatric institutions, subjected to pharmacological regimes that often do not have any impact on the course of the symptoms.

The healers themselves differentiate between a psychiatric illness and the calling. A primary difference is that the initiate who has a true calling is able to function optimally, with moments of disruption when the calling makes its presence felt, without losing conscious awareness. With a psychiatric illness, the effects are mostly pervasive, the patient's adaptive functioning is compromised and contact is lost with external reality. As Eliade (1989) noted, it is crucial to distinguish between a man possessed by archetypal content and in need of treatment and "a shaman or medicine man who knows how to control spirits and can give them free reign to work their powers without becoming possessed himself" (pp. 5–6).

Initiation symbolism can be found in most mythologies, indigenous belief systems, fairy tales, and biblical stories. This is an image of the archetypal pattern that weaves the covenant between man and God, between the ego and the Self, and is often accompanied by the psychological

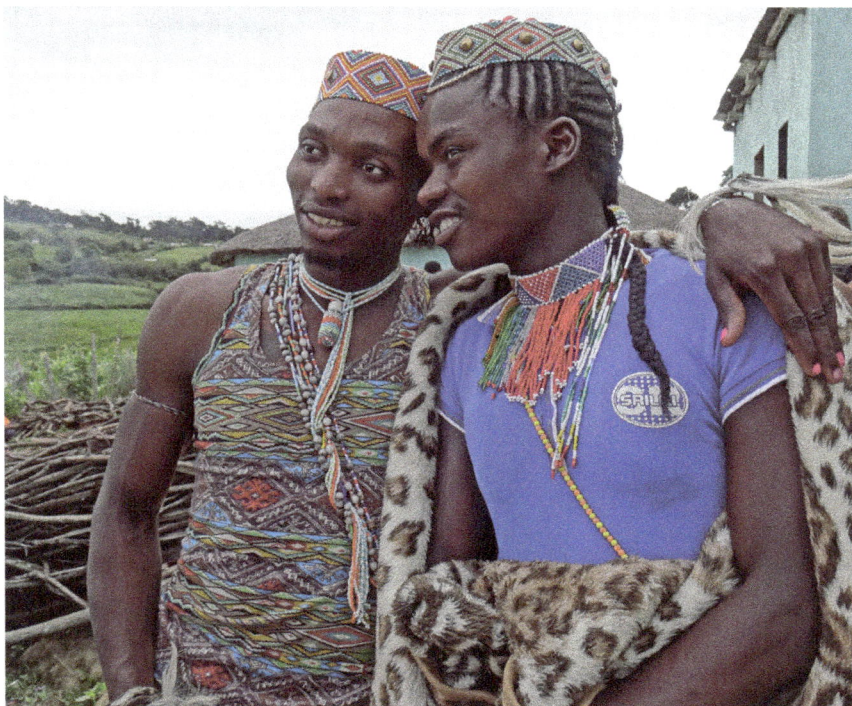

Figure 15: Two healers dressed in the individual regalia attend an initiation

imperative to honor the inner authority. These tales and myths often warn of dangerous reprisals if the call is refused. The initiation symbolism heralds the individuation process that births a reconciliation of opposites, of opposing forces.

Psychologically, during the *ukuthwasa* illness, the consciousness of the individual can be seen as becoming momentarily overwhelmed by the contents of the unconscious. This often results in vivid and disturbing dreams, confusion, disorientation, and feelings of alienation and isolation. Often such a feeling of crisis and dissolution indicates a need for a change in the attitude of ego consciousness, the resultant emergence of the Self, and a call for the reconciliation of opposites. From the African healing perspective, the disorientation as a result of the dreams requires the resolution of the *ukuthwasa* illness. This similarity between the *ukuthwasa* illness and psychological distress extends to the idea that both require a transformation of a life crisis. For the African healer this is achieved by attending to the needs of the ancestral spirits; psychologically, this is achieved by attending to the demands of the unconscious (Vera Buhrmann, personal communication, Aug. 8, 1984). As Ntombi commented, "the *ukuthwasa* sickness is really a soul sickness. When you are not connected to your ancestors, your soul is lost."

The acceptance of the *ukuthwasa* illness is often resisted for a number of reasons. On the outer level the resistance is connected to the physical demands of the treatment and training, which is long, demanding, and will interfere with other duties and relationships. The life of the healer is an onerous one, filled with difficulty as healers have to serve the ancestors, and their responsibilities are considerable. However, prolonged resistance to accepting the calling often results in further illness and psychological disturbances. As a healer explained:

> It is very demanding. There are lots of restrictions. Things you have to do and things you cannot do. You have to know how to behave, and the training is very difficult. You are away from home for long periods of time, and the *sangomas* are very strict. But I was happy to accept my calling. All my pain went away. I have not consulted a Western doctor for many years. Now when I have pain, I know it is about someone else. I feel their pain [people who need healing] in my body.

On an inner level, as noted, the terror and conflict that most initiates describe can be understood as the terror of facing the Godhead, the resolution of which will require an inner reconciliation. Psychologically, this resistance seems to be the fear of the numinous and the paradoxical nature of God. Jung (1952a) commented that "the paradoxical nature of God . . . tears man asunder into opposites and delivers him over to a seemingly insoluble conflict" (para. 738).

In Jungian analysis, as in many depth psychological intervention processes, the potential harm in not addressing psychological conflicts is apparent. One is frequently driven to enter into analysis by an unconscious inner conflict or an intolerable life situation, not only by rational or conscious choice. One has to make considerable sacrifices in order to undergo analysis or embark on analytical training. On the rational conscious level, analysands and patients often express an unwillingness or resistance to exploring the irrational symbolic world, which can be experienced as overwhelming and foreign. However, the inner compulsion is usually so strong that one feels as though one has little, if any, real choice. As von Franz reminds us:

> The initial encounter with the Self casts a dark shadow . . . as if the "inner friend" comes at first like a trapper to catch the helplessly struggling ego in his snare. . . . The hidden purpose of the oncoming darkness is generally something so unusual, so unique and unexpected, that . . . one can find out what it is only by means of dreams and fantasies welling up from the unconscious. (Quoted in Jung, 1990, p. 167)

The Stages of the *Ukuthwasa* Initiation

Healers describe the purpose of the *ukuthwasa* initiation as "the process of becoming a healer yourself." The neophyte is required to have a dream in which his or her teacher is revealed. The chosen teacher is further required to have dreamed of the initiate who will seek out assistance. Once the calling has been authenticated, the initiate then lives with the senior healer who becomes a mentor. At this time, the authenticity of the calling is repeatedly tested and confirmed through various rituals. Most importantly, the healer will attend carefully to the dreams of the initiate as well as to his or her own dreams about the initiate in order to guide the course of the initiation.

The procedures and ceremonies that characterize the *ukuthwasa* process do not end once the initiate has completed the training but rather continue to form a repeated integrative whole that is reentered time and again, each time with ever-increasing complexity, depth of meaning, and experience. The development of the healer is thus an ongoing lifelong process that is said to continue even after physical death.

The *ukuthwasa* initiation follows a recognizable pattern. There are four identifiable stages to this initiation process. The progression from one stage to the next is determined by pivotal dreams, and the duration of each stage is individual, depending on the proficiency of the initiate. At times one stage can last for a number of years. The completion of a stage is marked by a ceremony, which includes the ritual animal sacrifice. Each ceremony unfolds

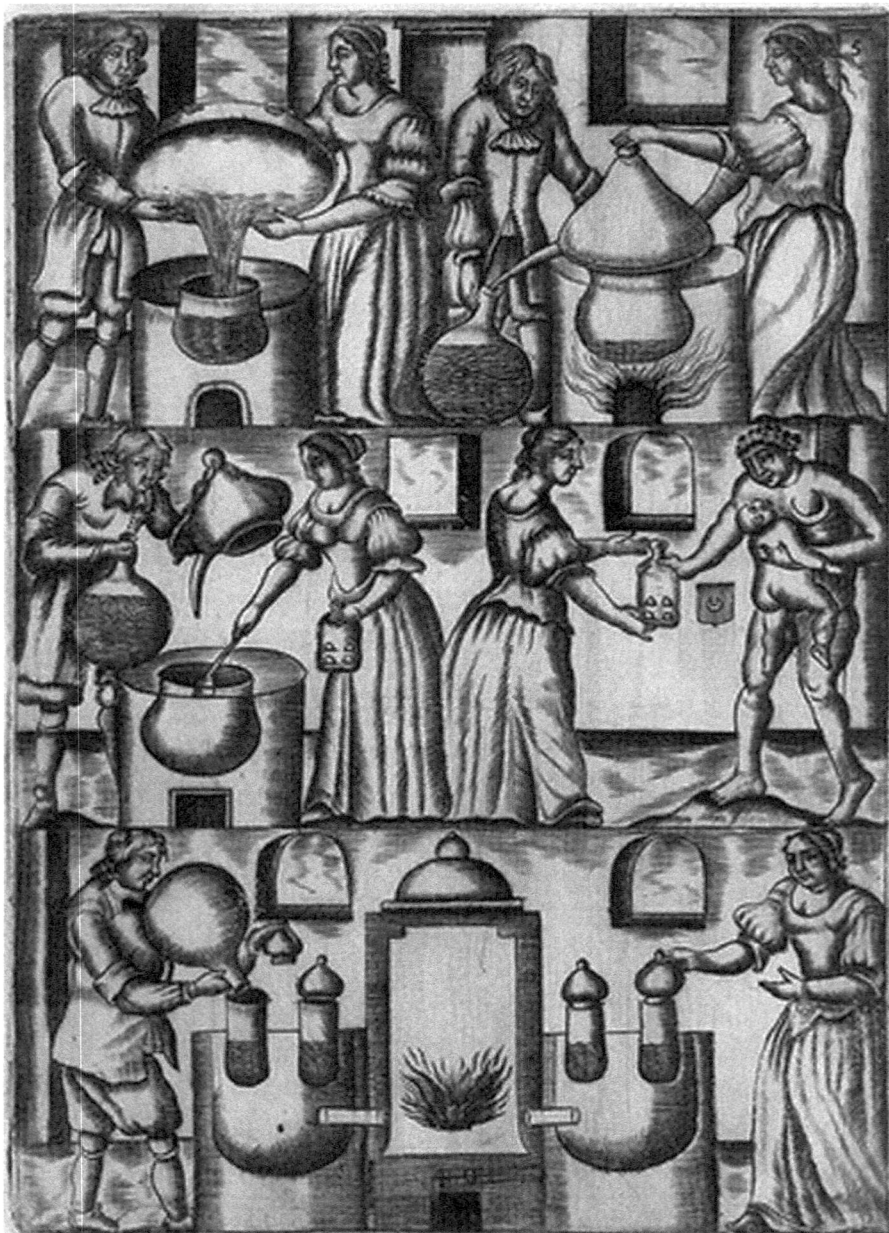

Figure 16. The alchemists at work depicting stages of the alchemical process of distillation and purification. Mutus Liber[11], plate 5

over a specified number of days and features changes to the color of the initiate's outer regalia.

The beginning of the *ukuthwasa* initiation illness is characterized by a period of blackness and despair. This is followed by a stage of whitening or an emergence from the darkness that heralds the beginning of the initiation process and the identification of the authenticity of the calling. In some initiatory processes there is an intermediate yellowing phase marked by the embodiment of the ritual teachings. The final phase of the initiation is the reddening stage, which culminates with the donning of the healer's regalia. At this time, the initiate is considered to have gained a level of proficiency to perform healings and to initiate novices. The successful resolution of this stage is marked by a graduation ceremony and the introduction of the qualified healer into the ranks of the healers.

In juxtaposition, the stages of the *ukuthwasa* initiation seems to mirror those of the alchemical stages elucidated so carefully by Jung, and they stand as a testimony to the archetypal patterns characteristic of deep creative unfolding of the unconscious psyche. As such the amplification of the different stages of the alchemical opus with the *ukuthwasa* initiation is appropriate here.

The alchemical opus, as described by Jung (1944), has four distinct stages: the *nigredo*, the *albedo*, the *citrinitas*, and the *rubedo*. Each stage is associated with the colors black, white, yellow, and red, respectively. The symbolism of the different colors is suggestive of the role color has in nature is an indication of transformation. Changes in color indicate a change in status. Fruit changes color when it ripens, animals indicate levels of fertility with color changes in plumage, and changes in mood are related to colors as are changes in the state of the soul. In addition, there are various alchemical operations, such as *mortificatio, sublimatio, solutio, coagulatio,* and *calcinatio* that are identifiable as operating throughout each of these stages. Jung (1977) gave a concise summary of the alchemical opus:

Alchemy represents the projection of a drama both cosmic and spiritual . . . right at the beginning you meet the "dragon" the chthonic spirit . . . or as the alchemists called it, the blackness, the *nigredo,* and this encounter produces suffering . . . Matter suffers right up to the final disappearance of the blackness, in psychological terms; the soul finds itself in the throes of melancholy, locked in the struggle with the "shadow." The mystery of the *coniunctio*, the central mystery of alchemy, aims precisely at the synthesis of opposites, the assimilation of the blackness . . . the *nigredo*. . . . In the language of the alchemists, matter suffers until the *nigredo* disappears when the "dawn" . . . will be announced . . . and new day will break . . . the *albedo*. But in this state of "white-ness" one does not live . . . it is a sort of abstract ideal state. In order to make it come alive, it must have "blood" . . . the *rubedo*, the "redness" of life . . . which . . . rejoins the profound unity of the psyche. Then the opus magnum is finished: the human soul is completely integrated. (p. 228)

It is interesting that here Jung does not mention the stage of the *citrinitas*. In *Psychology and Alchemy* (1944), Jung commented that the stage

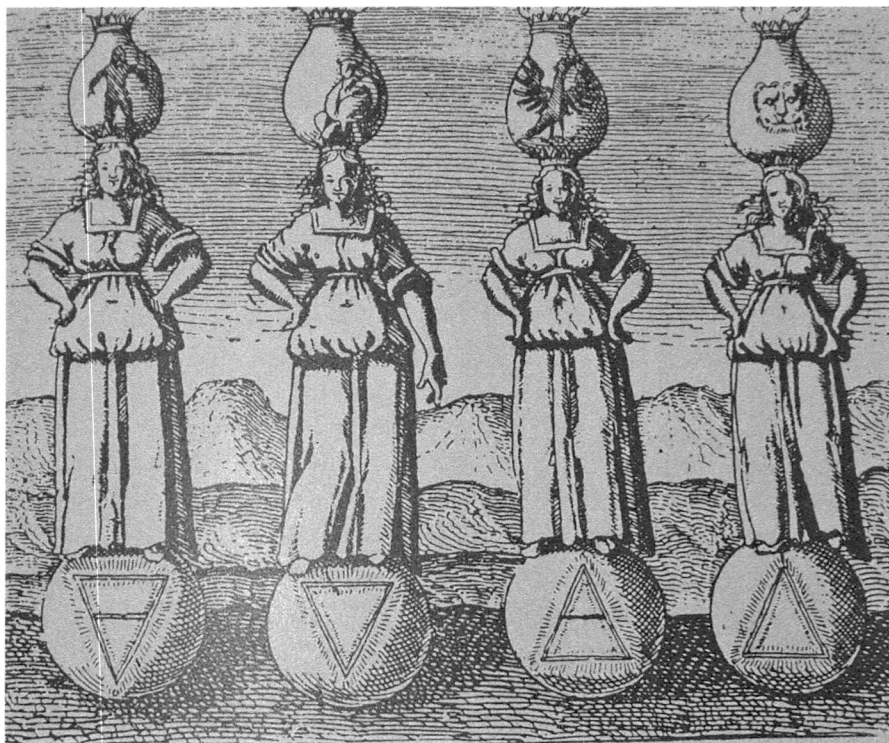

Figure 17. The four stages of the alchemical process.
The four elements are indicated on the balls

of the *citrinitas* may have belonged to an earlier formulation of the alchemical process (see chapter 7).

Jung (1944) noted that the stages of the alchemical opus echo the stages of the archetypal experience of individuation. Edinger (1991) reminds us that the origin of the term *psychotherapy* implies "to heal in the service of the gods . . . the service of the psyche" (p. 2). And further in relation to the role of alchemy, Edinger continued with the observation that "what makes alchemy so valuable for psychotherapy is that its images concretize the experiences of transformation" (1991, p. 2). For African healers, this would mean being in the service of the ancestors.

It is essential to be aware that these stages are not necessarily linear or discrete but rather unfold in a circular or spiral pattern, with many circumambulations within each stage. Reaching one level does not always lead to the next. Identifying the calling does not imply that the initiate will complete the training. The successful completion of the initiation can be interrupted by inflations, attempts to fast-track the process, or a disregard for the dreams or ancestral messages. These stages paralleled Ntombi's initiation in both the analytical vessel and the realm of the healer, as described in the following chapters.

Chapter 5
Imithi Emnyama:
The Black Medicine

You start off with an illness, unhappiness . . . you just get more
and more sick. I almost lost my mind.
—Ntombi

The *ukuthwasa* illness, as described in the previous chapter, bears remarkable similarity to certain Western diagnostic criteria for psychopathology and is characterized by vivid, repetitive, and often disturbing dreams. Within the African healing cosmology the presence of such dreams takes precedence over other symptoms. As we have seen, the African healer ascribes to dreams a value and meaning that parallels the importance given to dreams in Jungian psychology. The dream is the primary channel of communication with and from the ancestor as it was for Jung with and from the unconscious psyche. For the healer, "the dream is to see the truth at night." After the first session, Ntombi reported the following initial dream (see also Radomsky, 2009):

> I am back at home, in my grandparent's home, the home where I was born. I am sitting in the middle of the doorway to the kraal. But the kraal is square, no longer round. The animals come towards me, the chickens and goats and cows. Many, many of them, they come towards me and they will not stop. I cannot get away, there is nowhere to go. I sit looking terrified at the animals, fearing that they will trample me. There's something wrong with them too, they are all monstrous: the goats have chicken's heads, the cows have goat's heads. It's all wrong and I force myself to wake up.

This dream had a profound effect on Ntombi, propelling her to seek assistance and convincing her of the reality of the objective psyche. She had previously resisted the encounter with the unconscious; as she had paid no heed to the call from the psyche, the dream forced her to reconsider. Jung taught that the initial dream is an important dream that often hints at the entire analytical process. I was concerned with this dream as the lysis of the dream seemed uncertain and ambivalent. I was also curious as I had in mind a dream of mine from night before Ntombi's first appointment. It seemed to me my dream might be relevant to her process and may offer a compensatory image to her distress. I dreamed:

> I am driving in a city and I get lost. The roads lead me into a rural area of natural bush and open grasslands. Large white goats roam the area. At a low rise where two roads intersect is a huge tree. I am now on foot and I walk around the tree behind which is a clearing. In the clearing is a group of healers. I am intrigued by the beautiful intricate beadwork of their regalia. The healers are performing a ritual ceremony and an old woman calls me over to assist. I am then in my own garden and I am busy planting new seedlings. A black woman comes to the gate and asks me if I will help her plant her seeds.

From the perspective of the *ukuthwasa* tradition, Ntombi's dream served several functions. The dream indicated the cause of her depression, her illness, in that the dream imagery is indicative of her need to accept a calling and to begin the initiatory process symbolized by the visitation of the animals, in particular, chickens, goats, and cows. These three animals refer to the sacrificial animals that form part of the initiatory ceremonies and herald different stages of the novice's accomplishments on her path to becoming the fully trained healer (at times, the bull replaces the cow as one of the sacrificial animals, see chapter 7).

The beginning of the *ukuthwasa* illness is a time usually experienced as one in which all usual ways of being no longer hold, resulting in the darkening characterized by feelings of blackness, depression, alienation, and isolation. Ntombi described a time of intense suffering accompanied by treatment-resistant physical and psychological symptoms.

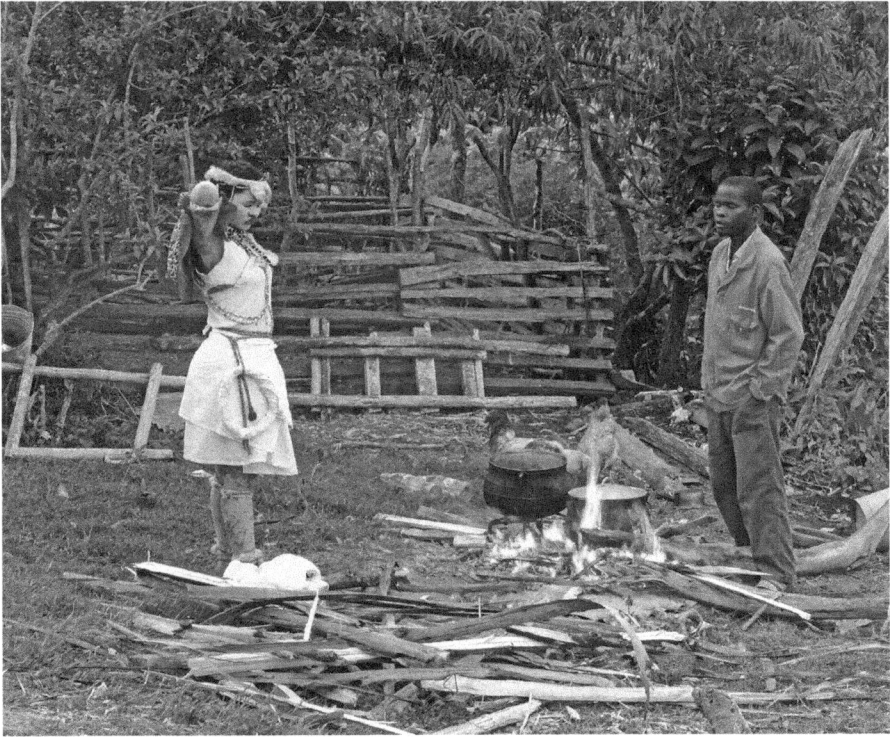

Figure 18. An initiate prepares for the early morning ritual

This is akin to the *nigredo*, the individual *metanoia*, characterized by a turning away from the outer and turning inward. Psychologically, this is a dark night of the soul, a state of disorientation, exhaustion, self-doubt, and inertia. A time of shadow, but in which, as Jung (1944) explained, perhaps lies the psyche's illimitable potential and the germ of the golden embryo of the Self. As Jung (1952b) highlighted: "The alchemists sought their *prima materia* in the excrement . . . from which it was hoped, the mystic figure of the *filius philosophorum* would emerge" (para. 276).[12] The healers refer to this stage of the initiatory illness as being without light and in the darkness.

Psychologically, this corresponds to that phase of therapy that requires reductive work: delving into past traumas and conflicts. The aim is to evoke the realization that there is also something else at work in our lives, something beyond our personal control, something archetypal that influences and interferes with our personal conscious desires and needs, and challenges the ego position. This is also the difficult time of con-frontation with the shadow. Jung (1955-56) reminds us:

> Confrontation with the shadow produces at first a dead balance, a standstill that hampers moral decisions and makes convictions ineffective or even impossible. Everything becomes doubtful, which is why the alchemists called this stage the *nigredo*, *tenebrositas*, chaos, melancholia. It is right that the magnum opus should begin at this point. (para. 708)

The Alchemical *Mortificatio*

The alchemical *mortificatio* is the central operation of the *nigredo* or the blackening and refers to an experience of death. Edinger (1991) noted that the "*mortificatio* is the most negative operation in alchemy. It has to do with darkness, defeat, torture, mutilation, death, and rotting which ultimately in turn leads to growth and resurrection" (p. 148). Psychologically, the *mortificatio* has to do with a confrontation with the shadow, the first stage of the analytical work characterized by outbursts of affect, resentment, pleasure, and power. These primitive affects must all undergo a *mortifactio* if the primitive, infantile libido is to be transformed.

Images of putrefaction are characteristic of this stage, accompanied by a sense of hopelessness, darkness, where the light of the ego is eclipsed and falls into an experience of darkness. But the darkness often contains its compensatory opposite and out of the darkness a new dawn can emerge, as black is also the color of "resurrection and possible rejuvenation" or preparation for a renewal (Apt, 2005, p. 104). As Jung explained (1955–56):

> Everyone who becomes conscious of even a fraction of his unconscious gets outside his own time . . . into a kind of solitude . . . only there is it possible to meet the "god of salvation." Light is manifest in the darkness, and out of danger, the rescue comes. (para. 258)

The *nigredo* stage is experienced as a kind of deathlike state for ego consciousness and for everything that came before. In Jung's words, "the experience of the self is always a defeat for the ego" (1955–56, para. 778). As Edinger (1991) explained:

> It is as though the psyche cannot come into existence as a separate entity until the death of the literal, the concrete, the physical. The collective unconscious is equivalent to the land of the dead or the afterlife, and a descent into the collective unconscious is called a *nekyia* because an encounter with the autonomous psyche is felt as a death of this world. (p. 163)

It is through the recognition and acceptance of the calling and the entry into the initiation that the neophyte experiences the possibility of a renewal and the emergence of something new. Eliade (1958) notes that the suffering and the solitude is part of the initiation process as "a symbolic return to chaos . . . equivalent to preparing a new creation" (p. 89). This experience of a renewal or a resurrection can be understood psychologically as an awakening to a higher state of consciousness. Within the African healing modality this awakening results in the acquisition of healing abilities. From the illness that characterizes the *ukuthwasa* process, potentially a neophyte is born.

Thus the identification of the calling through the *ukuthwasa* illness is characterized by a deep state of depression, darkness, and dissolution. This is experienced as a disaster by the individual ego but also can herald the moment of potential when a new symbol of the Self may be born. But at this threshold of healing and transformation, there is also the greatest crisis and difficulty, as occurs in analysis when the person recognizes the difficulty of letting go of a neurotic attitude. As Ntombi described:

> I saw it in my father. He was always depressed and angry. Everyone was scared of him. He had the calling. He should have been a healer, but the church told him it was a bad thing, so he never answered the call, and he died an unhappy man. I got it then. I was depressed all the time. I used to cry a lot. I recognized the tears were a symbol of something, something pushing from inside. There was this big gap, an emptiness in my heart. This was the beginning, before my calling was recognized.

The *nigredo* is further symbolized by the distortions of the animals in Ntombi's dream, which seem to warn her of the danger in continuing to resist the calling, and are also reflective of her own distorted outer identity. Marie-Louise von Franz (1997a) has noted that the ego can focus on adaptation, and neglect unconscious material, which may be inappropriate for conscious adaption. The ego thus adopts one-sidedness that is not in accord with the instinctive totality. The distortions of the animals in Ntombi's dream are perhaps also reflective of something psychic that does not as yet know what it wants to become. This is indicative of a conscious lack of discernment, wherein there is as yet no appropriate vehicle in the consciousness for the dreamer to express the distorting effects of autonomous or unconscious complexes. Von Franz (1997a) spoke of monsters in dreams as amorphous primal deities, frightful, unapproachable, and incomprehensible. The ego experiences its formlessness or distortions as something inhuman and hostile.

Archetypally, the distortions reflect the ambivalent nature of the alchemical Mercurius. Mercurius is the preeminent symbol for the mysterious substance of transformation, a symbol of the unconscious psyche itself, consisting of all the possible opposites, both matter and spirit. A psychopomp but also darkness, spirit and its antagonist, which carries as Jung (1944) discerned, "the lowest *prima materia* and highest *lapis philosophorum*" (para. 84).

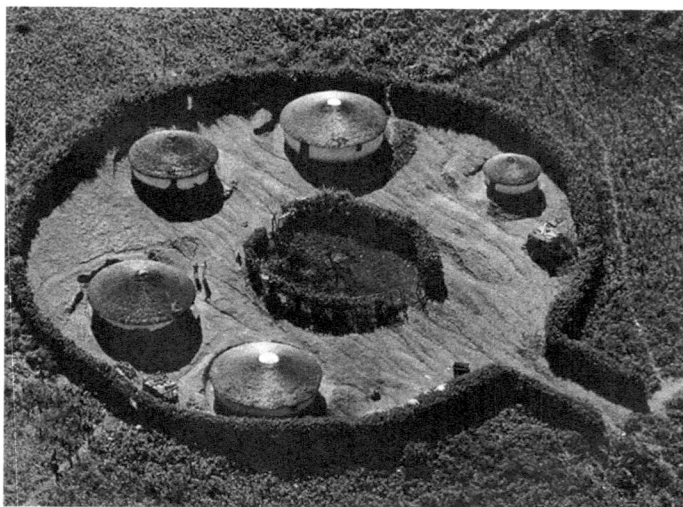

Figure 19. An aerial view of a traditional Zulu kraal, Kwa-Zulu, Natal

The location of the dream in the family kraal is an important detail. The kraal is the heart of the traditional rural homestead. The center of the kraal is where the cattle are penned. This is functional in that it ensures the safety of the cattle, the wealth of the homestead. Psychologically, the cattle, symbolic of an aspect of the instinctive nature, are housed in the center of the kraal, the seat of the ancestors. Thus the kraal in the dream seems symbolic of the need for Ntombi to return home to her birthplace and the place of the ancestors—psychologically, a return to the Self. Once the Self is constellated, if its impulse is refused by the ego, it can turn dangerously negative, resulting in illness and misfortune, which reflects the psychological understanding of the wrath of the ancestors. Once the Self is activated through the calling, individuation must proceed.

The image of the square kraal in the dream requires amplification. Characteristically the kraal is circular, both in its overall formation and in each individual hut within the kraal. The kraal evokes the image of the temenos, a magic protective circle or enclosure. It is here that the dreamer finds herself rooted, unable to move. This is symbolic of the prison from which there is no escape, but also of the creative womb. Jung (1944) taught that this central circular formation is symbolic of "the seeding place where the diamond body, the integrated personality is produced" (para. 170). The round kraal and fence delimit the field of the temenos inside which the dreamer is solitary, in her own center and at the center, which is also the sacred place of the ancestors. It is here that the archetypal world, in the form of the distorted animals, breaks in, manifest in its numinosity and demanding attention. It is perhaps positive that Ntombi is contained within the sacred circle wherein transformation can occur. As Eliade (1958) noted, "the place becomes . . . a source of power and sacredness and enables whomever enters it to have a share in the power, to hold communion with the sacred" (p. 369).

The squaring of the kraal in the dream is reminiscent of the squaring of the circle, the division of wholeness into parts and into directions, eliciting the symbolism of the four. Here we find another image of the mandala (see chapter 3 and the healing dance ritual). As Jung (1955) highlights regarding the mandala symbolism:

> There are innumerable variants of the motif . . . but they are all based on the squaring of the circle. Their basic motive is the premonition of a centre of the personality, a kind of central point

within the psyche, to which everything is related, by which everything is arranged, and which is itself a source of energy. . . . This centre is not felt or thought of as the ego but, if one may so express it, as the *self.* (para. 634)

Jung (1955) further explained that "the 'squaring of the circle' is one of the many archetypal motifs which . . . can even be called the *archetype of wholeness*" (para. 715). The square is the fourfold structure that expresses totality with an emphasis on static, structural aspects, a symbol for earth. The circle is the original perfection, symbolizing eternity, the germ of the beginning in which opposites are in union, a symbol for the Godhead and the Self, the cycle of life, completion and heaven. Jung (1977) developed the importance of the mandala symbol when he stated:

The mandala . . . is what they call in alchemy the *quadrature circuli,* the square in the circle or the circle in the square. It is an age-old symbol that goes right back to the pre-history of man. It is found all over the earth and it expresses either the deity or the self. These two terms are psychologically very much related— which doesn't mean that I believe that God is the self or that the self is God. I simply state that there is a psychological relation between them. The mandala . . . expresses the fact that there is a centre and a periphery and it tries to embrace the whole . . . when during treatment there is a great disorder and chaos in a man's mind, this symbol can appear in the form of a mandala in a dream . . . The mandala appears spontaneously as a compensatory archetype . . . showing the possibility of order. (pg. 327)

Von Franz (1974) elaborated that the four is qualitatively connected to complete conscious orientation, the archetypal background by which ego consciousness is structured (p. 246). This is also a symbol of the emerging consciousness, where the dream ego awakens to the numinosity of the unconscious.

Edinger (1995) commented that the circling of the square and the squaring of the circle is a preoccupation with "an innate archetypal yearning for individuation" (p. 199). He goes on to explain that at birth "the circle would represent the condition of initial unconscious unity" (p. 200). With psychological growth and ego development, the square emerges as a symbol of the emergence of consciousness and "the discrimination of the four functions" (p. 200). With further development, these four elements are united and the circle returns as a symbol of "wholeness . . . on a conscious level" (p. 201). Edinger further elucidated:

> Paradise can be understood . . . in terms of the circle-square-circle sequence. Paradise is the first circle, the state of original wholeness. The full development of the ego as an earthly material manifestation would be the square . . . with the second circle, the four elements are unified into the quintessence and the state of original wholeness returns on the conscious level. (1995, p. 201)

Ntombi's fear is understandable in the face of these numinous creatures. To meet them outside of the temenos would be to encounter them where danger lay, the danger of inflations and possible psychosis. The significance of the temenos is exactly that of a protective circle inside which the dreamer can potentially endure the manifestation of the numinosum, which protects against the risk of dissociation of the personality by the influx of archetypal forces.

The alchemical prescription of keeping the vessel closed as she sits, unable to do anything but contemplate her fate at the entrance to the sacred enclosure, reflects, too, the meaning of the word *contemplation* (*con-templum*), a place regarded primarily as the dwelling place of the deity. It is here that she receives the visitation, where the unconscious psyche manifests and where she is confronted with a direct call from the unconscious to action. At this time Ntombi dreamed:

> *I'm at a family gathering. All my ancestors, living and dead are there: My great grandparents, grandfather, uncles, aunts, cousins. In the center of the gathering there is a young girl. She seems to be ill, in a lot of pain and someone tells me that she is deaf as well. An old man approached me. He tells me my task is to heal the girl so that she can hear.*

Psychologically, for Ntombi, this *nigredo* was indicative of old worn-out attitudes that required transformation. This included her neurotic insistence on her need to be white—her destructive use of skin lighteners and her rejection of her cultural heritage. The *nigredo* indicates the need for something to change, the need for a renewal or separation from the old worn-out unconscious identification, which often manifests in a state of confusion, a *massa confusa*. In the alchemical opus, the renewal begins with working on the *massa confusa* to bring consciousness to the confusion and to release the hold of the unconsciousness on the personality. As von Franz (1998) summarizes:

> In the first phase, the *nigredo*, the initial material (*prima materia*) is dissolved, calcinated, pulverized . . . The operator feels bewildered, disoriented, succumbs to a deep melancholy . . . the *nigredo* has its parallels in the individuation process, in the confrontation with the shadow. Everything which one has criticized, with moral indignation, in others, is "served up" in dreams as a part of one's own being . . . The ego feels robbed of its illusionary omnipotence and confronted with the dark and bewildering power of the unconscious. (pp. 222-223)

Ntombi's shift to the next stage of her initiation was suggested by the following dream:

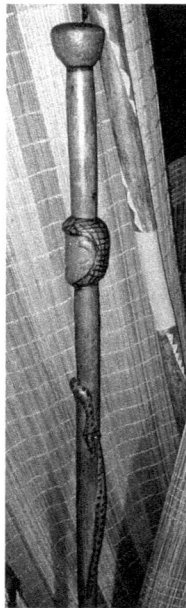

Figure 20: Carved stick used by healers

92

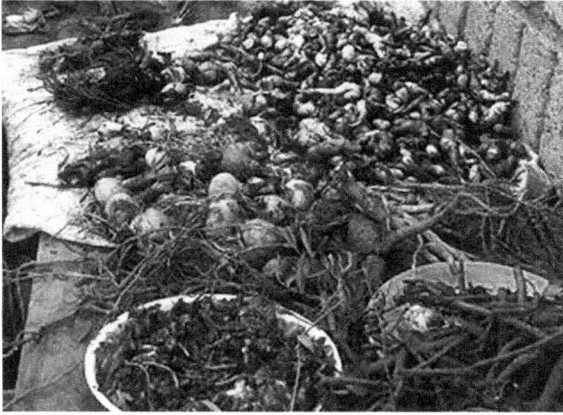

Figure 21. Black *muthi,* consisting of different indigenous herbs that function as purgatives

I'm lying at home. I have been very ill. At the doorway a man enters, he's carrying a beautifully carved stick made from dark ebony. He comes to where I am lying in my bed and gives me the stick. He says: "It's time to get up now".

The symbolism of the *nigredo*, the blackness, extends further with respect to the herbal remedies prepared at each stage. The medicinal herbs and *muthi* used during this first stage, the *nigredo* phase, are referred to by African healers as the *imithi emnyama* (black medicines). These are mostly purgatives, said to rid the body of the dark energies and to reestablish a balance both within and without.

The healer's constant reminders that this process cannot be fast-tracked is indicative of their intuitive awareness of the ebb and flow of psychic energies and the transformative power or effect that lies in the gradual engagement of consciousness with the unconscious, ego with the Self. Only then can the enantiodromia take place where the *nigredo*, the darkness, falls into its opposite: the *albedo,* the lightness and the associated dawning of consciousness.

Chapter 6
Imithi Emhlope:
The White Medicine

My spirit was crying out to be recognized,
but I did not know how to see the signs.
—Ntombi

Ntombi's need to acknowledge her calling and transition to the next stage of her initiation is illustrated in the following dream:

My grandfather who passed before comes to me. He is begging me to return home and to take up the mantle of the family ancestral healing line. He shows me how to take care of all his healing implements, which I must use and which must be buried. He explains in detail the process. He shows me how to mix all the herbs, some must be soaked in bowls of water, some are burnt, other dried. He explains how many animals must be sacrificed and how I must continue my learning to be a healer.

Ntombi dreamed further of her grandfather's regalia, which were lying in the homestead and which had not been ritually taken care of. These are unambiguous dream images that confirm the authenticity of her calling within the culture, in that the dream images seem to compensate for Ntombi's ego-driven resistance to accept her calling. Psychologically, the dreams herald the call for a return to the Self, to return home, to the original matrix from which she came. The call is an archetypal image that initiates individuation and births the awareness of a transpersonal other, a call to awaken and to remember one's heavenly origins.

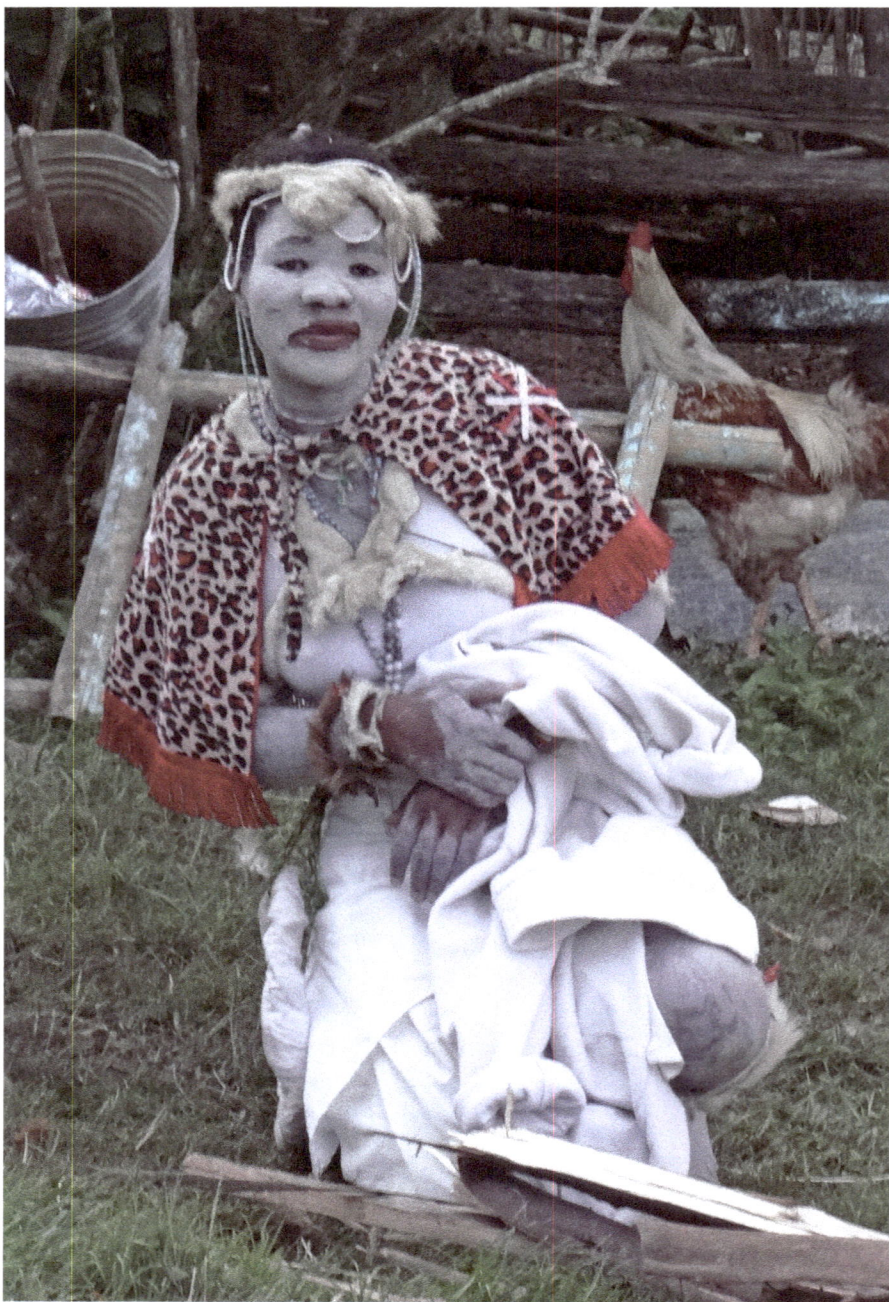

Figure 22. An initiate with white face paint and white regalia

The most obvious outer sign of this stage of the initiation is the color white. The neophyte's body and face is painted with white clay. Each initiate is required to wear white clothes and beads at all times. The donning of white clothes is found in many initiation systems across indigenous cultures, as well as in the healing incubations and initiations of ancient Greece, and evokes images of the acolytes in Buddhist temples or the aesthetics of the Christian tradition. According to C.A. Meier (1989), such white garb is said to represent a new identity and is also "the garment of the god, the indication of the appearance of god" (p. 87). White is the initiatory color that also suggests purity and the newborn. Von Franz (1997b) explained that in psychological language the color white has "to do with the remotest depths of the unconscious, where it has become almost abstract" (p. 49). White, as the color that reflects all colors, is further associated with purity, immortality, and life transitions, both with respect to birth and death (Apt, 2005).

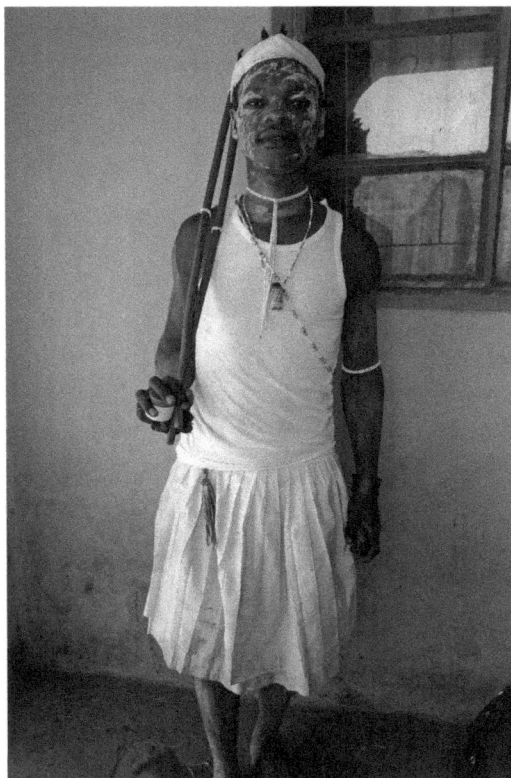

Figure 23. Male initiate during the whitening stage

African healers explain that white is a time of new birth, innocence, and humility, symbolizing a state of transition and the potential for the emergence of something new. During this stage the *thwasa* is referred to as imbued with *ukuhanya*, or light. This stage can be likened to the emergence of a new awareness after the darkening, as Jung (1946b) noted: "the whitening (*albedo*) is likened to the *ortus solis*, the sunrise; it is the light; the illumination that follows the darkness" (para. 484).

During this time of the whitening or *albedo* stage of the *ukuthwasa* process, each novice leaves home and goes to live with the healers. All outer signs of ego identification are removed, and the *thwasa* is seen as faceless, unborn, and without an identity. The novice is nameless. Her face is painted white, devoid of individual character, in essence creating a mask, no shoes are worn, and foods are restricted. No sugars are allowed nor are any products of the sacrificial animals that participate in the future rituals. Outer distractions are minimized and all activities are in service of the Self. Most importantly, it is a time of strict celibacy.

With the acceptance of her calling, Ntombi moved out of her city home to go live with the healer who would continue her training. As the *thwasa*, she was required to serve the experienced healers and to attend to their every need. Such is the synergy inherent in this relationship that the *thwasa* soon develops the ability to anticipate the needs of the healers and the homestead in which he or she lives at this time. An attitude and posture of deep humility is nurtured, and all attempts to assert oneself are discouraged. The healers explain that this is necessary as during this time the *thwasa* becomes aware of the connection to spirit without the interference of ego needs or desires, in psychological terms, the withdrawal of projections. The rational questioning mind is stilled, characterized by a state of becoming quiet, more detached, and more objective. This is an essential state from which to approach the unconscious in order that the deeper layers of the psyche, in the form of ancestral communications, can be accessed.

This stage of the *ukuthwasa* experience, which the initiates describe as difficult, demanding, and isolating but also liberating, is likened to the alchemical task of refining and separating the *prima materia* of ego-Self identity, so that the Self can be freed from the contamination of the ego attitudes that may be contrary to the development of consciousness. There is a cessation of outer activities, and everything is put into the retort before a synthesis can begin that will herald the next stage. In the initiation system, the emergence from the period of isolation and darkness is signified by the *ukuhlamba*, rituals of purification, purging, and washing. The healers explain that these rituals instill in the initiate a state of purity and clarity in order to be receptive to the communications from the ancestors. Marie-Louise von Franz (1980a) noted that

> the great effort and trouble continues from the *nigredo* to the *albedo*; that is said to be the hard part . . . The *nigredo*—the blackness, the terrible depression and state of dissolution—has to be compensated by the hard work of the alchemist and that the hard work consists, amongst other things, in constant washing. (p. 220)

Psychologically, as von Franz explained, the action of washing is akin to the "cleaning up" of projections and conscious attitudes. This entails

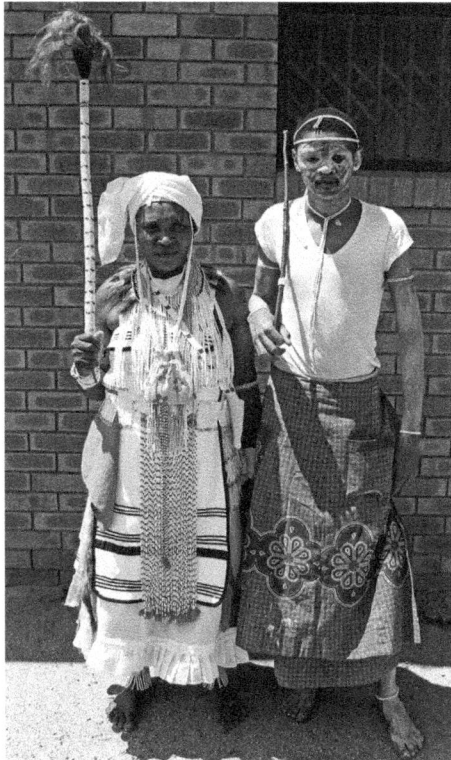

Figure 24. An initiate and his teacher with the white beads of the whitening stage

recognizing aspects of the shadow that are unconscious and often projected onto another. Here the cleaning of the projections would mean recollecting that which has been projected and integrating the projection into the personality, thereby enhancing individual conscious awareness. Through hard work, the darkness of the *nigredo* lightens, becoming white, the *albedo* corresponding to a deep introversion and the withdrawal of projections.

The Alchemical *Sublimatio* and *Solutio*

The alchemical operations of the *sublimatio* and *solutio* are applicable at this stage. *Sublimatio* pertains to air and the volatizing of matter. During the *albedo* phase of the *ukuthwasa* initiation, the neophyte is expected to forego all earthly pleasures and comforts, in effect, spiritualizing ego needs and desires and rising above the bodily needs, the concrete. This is a time of physical celibacy in order to transfer energy from external, profane matters, to rise above earthly restraints, and to foster the connection to the unconscious, the ancestors, and the spiritual. Jung (1973) explained that "*sublimatio* is part of the royal art where the true gold is made" (p. 171). It is the extraction process whereby spirit is released from matter.

The *sublimatio* is often associated with purification, where matter and spirit are separated and purified. It requires certain detachment from earthly matters and contains the dangers of psychic dissociation or inflation. It embodies a movement farther away from the personal, farther away from earthbound daily reality. The initiate is removed from his or her usual life routines, gives up all outer signs of individuality or identity, and spends the time in a state of deep introversion.

The operation *solutio* forms a central aspect to the alchemical work and refers to the element of water symbolizing the liquefaction of solids and a return to the state of undifferentiated matter or the *prima materia*. As Edinger (1991) exemplified, "water was thought of as the womb and the *solutio* as a return to the womb for rebirth" (p. 47). This, according to alchemical treatises, was a precondition for transformation. During the white phase of the *ukuthwasa* initiation, the rituals that the neophyte undergoes, in addition to the requirements and restrictions noted above, involve the processes of washing, bathing, and purifying. The healers explain that this aims to reduce and refine the personality and to return it to a state of pre-

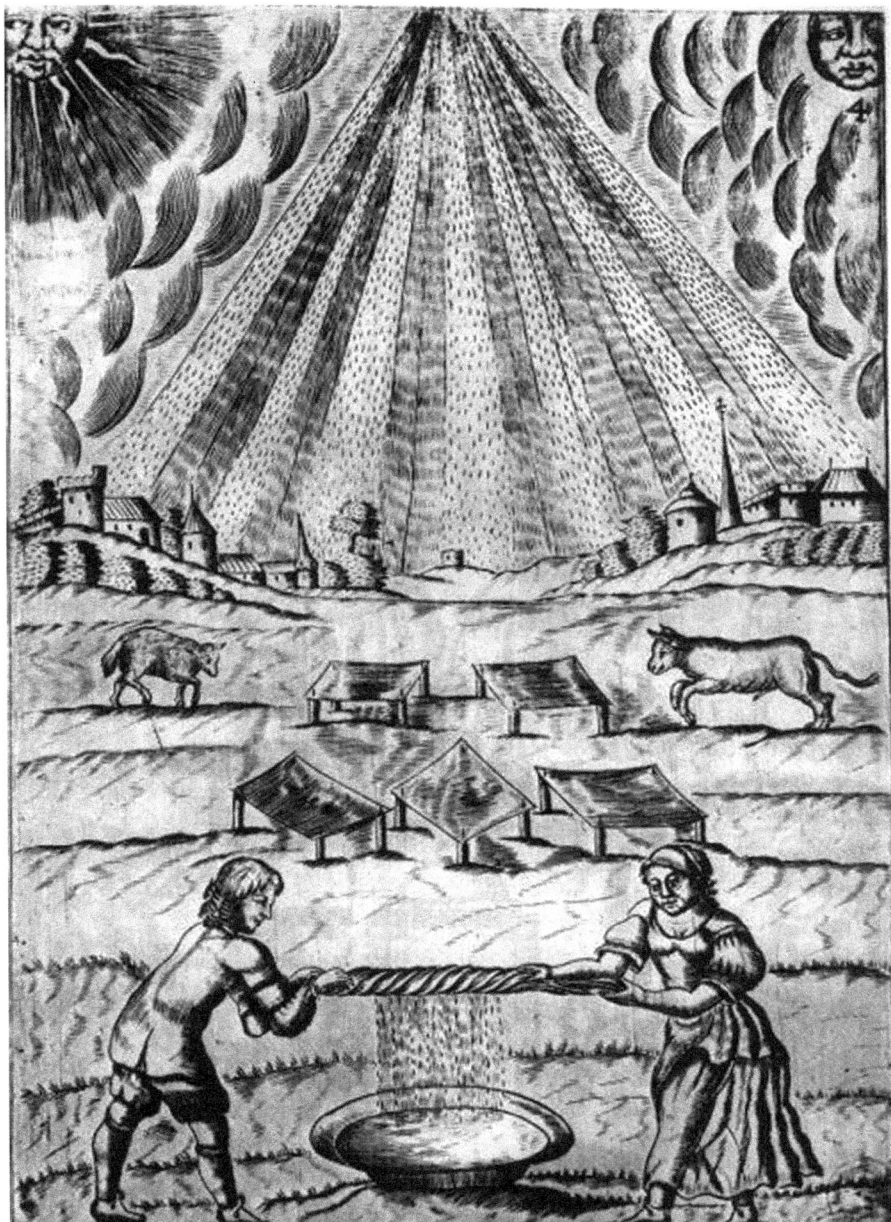

Figure 25. Two alchemists at work engaged in wringing out the washing symbolizing the purification and cleansing stage of the process. Mutus liber, pl. 4

birth purity in order for the initiate to acquire the capacities of flexibility and elasticity, and to nurture the relationship to the ancestral communications.

As in analysis, the fixed or rigid ego states or attitudes are dissolved by attending to the messages from the unconscious in order for change to occur. The initiate's experience of this stage is often frightening and very difficult, as the usual ego states are no longer applicable and the new state of the healer has yet to be born; thus, it can also be experienced as a kind of *mortificatio,* as described above. Edinger (1991) noted: "that which is being dissolved will experience that *solutio* as an annihilation of itself . . . however the *solutio* leads to an emergence of a rejuvenated new form" (p. 52). As such, the rituals are very specific with many restrictions in order to contain the experience of dissolution and disintegration. Jung (1955–56) commented that "everyone who becomes conscious of even a fraction of his unconscious gets outside of his own time . . . into a kind of solitude . . . but only then is it possible to meet the gods" (para. 258). This is the time for dissolving attitudes that have become hardened and stagnant and is followed in a later stage by the "fixing," or stabilizing, those that are unformed and uncertain, a period alchemically referred to as *solve et coagula*.

An important aspect of the initiation and related to the *albedo* phase is the healer-initiate relationship, which mirrors analyst-analysand relationship in many respects. Here, the initiate encounters in the healer a more integrated personality, and the initiate experiences this relationship as being swallowed up by the healer in order to transform. As noted, it is not uncommon for the healer to dream about the initiate's process. The healers describe their awareness that they have a communication with the unconscious of the initiate and vice versa. At this time, a connection between the healer and the initiate develops, which is reminiscent of Jung's ideas about the transference and countertransference.

Von Franz (1998) explains that the *albedo* phase in analysis heralds the emergence of the problem of the integration of the contra-sexual components in the individuation process; the anima in the case of men and the animus in the case of women.[13] The healer-initiate dyad is often a contra-sexual couple, not unlike the alchemists who were predominantly men and who worked with their female counterpart or *soror mystica*. In the alchemical symbolism this is represented by the mystic marriage (see chapter 9 and 10).

The whitening stage of the *ukuthwasa* initiation, or the progression from the *nigredo* to the *albedo*, can continue for some time, often years. It is a circular progression, often returning again and again to another *nigredo*. The neophyte is faced with the task of challenging ego desires and expectations and learning to defer to another authority. This is externally projected first onto the senior healers and later, if this process is successfully navigated, onto the inner authority symbolized by the inner voice of the ancestors. It is an arduous and demanding stage, and many do not proceed further.

The *albedo* is experienced as a release from the dark tortuous *nigredo* but remains a state of not yet a fully embodied renewal. The old neurotic attitudes do not let go easily and carry their own energy, often unconsciously or compulsively. The letting go of old worn-out attitudes is often experienced as a death, followed by a certain limbo state of not being. This is beautifully demonstrated in the characteristics of the whitening stage. The healers refer to the whitening as the "as yet unborn" state, a suspended animation, so to say, a realization that the old no longer serves the personality, but the new is not yet clear. At this time an awareness of the autonomous unconscious psyche is paramount for the novice and the new developing ego attitude, lest despair swamp the fragile new realization. It is the stage where the healer's support is most notable.

The healers possessed a natural awareness of what was needed in order to facilitate the shift from the *nigredo* to the *albedo*. This stage of the initiatory process seemed carefully orchestrated to serve and reinforce the retort and to guide the psychic energy toward an inner transformation. The *albedo*, for the alchemists, was a time of spiritualization, as it is for the initiate. The neophyte exists in a state of aesthetic humility, celibacy, following a restrictive mode of living, focused on psychological aspects, the development of the awareness of an inner authority, and the ego's relationship with respect to this authority.

The healers acknowledge that the *thwasa* is vulnerable to inflation or despair at this stage, in which levels of previously unconscious identifications and projections are stripped away. The healers maintain a strict parental stance toward the novice and seem to function as an auxiliary ego, much like in analysis. The healers, too, are vulnerable to inflations as the novice's devotion is complete. I reflected on the limitations of the analytical container in this regard. Analysis is usually conducted in discrete hourly sessions, once or twice in the week. The analyst typically has little direct knowledge of the life of the analysand outside of the therapeutic hour other than that which the analysand chooses to share. My experience of the two processes, the initiation container versus the analytical container, brought home the need for this container to remain absolute. But also, the notion of the Western-based adherence to the analytical hour as distinct from the life of the analysand brings unique limitations. In my work with Ntombi, my Western-based training with respect to professional boundaries stood in stark contrast to the inclusion of each initiate in the life of the healer and how this actually facilitated the development of the novice to a dramatic extent.

The pendulous movement of the transition from *nigredo* to *albedo* reminds us how difficult it is for ego consciousness to humble itself sufficiently to be aware that it is not in control and to relate to the Self. Old attitudes hold fast and must be dissolved and sacrificed akin to the sacrifice of certainty of the complex or neurosis and the ego's position as the center of the personality. Dismemberment is characteristic of this stage as outdated attitudes are stripped away to give way to a renewal, which also means tolerating uncertainty and not knowing (the theme of dismemberment returns in a later aspect of the initiation in chapter 9). At this time, Ntombi shared the following dream:

I am lying out on a ledge in a remote region. It is semi-dark, like just before the sunrise. I am aware of being quite paralyzed, unable to move. A large bird hovers above me. It dives down to attack me, over and over. It's as if parts of my body are torn apart.

Jung (1955–56) explained the link between the alchemical *solutio* and the motif of dismemberment (para. 365). Citing Dorn, Jung elaborated that the dissolution required during the alchemical opus consists of "dissolution by dismemberment and pulverization" and essentially, the outcome of the dismemberment is rejuvenation.[14] Jung (1954e) elaborated:

Dismembering . . . corresponds to the idea of dividing the chaos into four elements . . . The purpose of the operation is to create the beginning of order in the *massa confusa* . . . The psychological parallel to this is the reduction to order, through reflection, of apparently chaotic fragments of the unconscious. (para. 111)

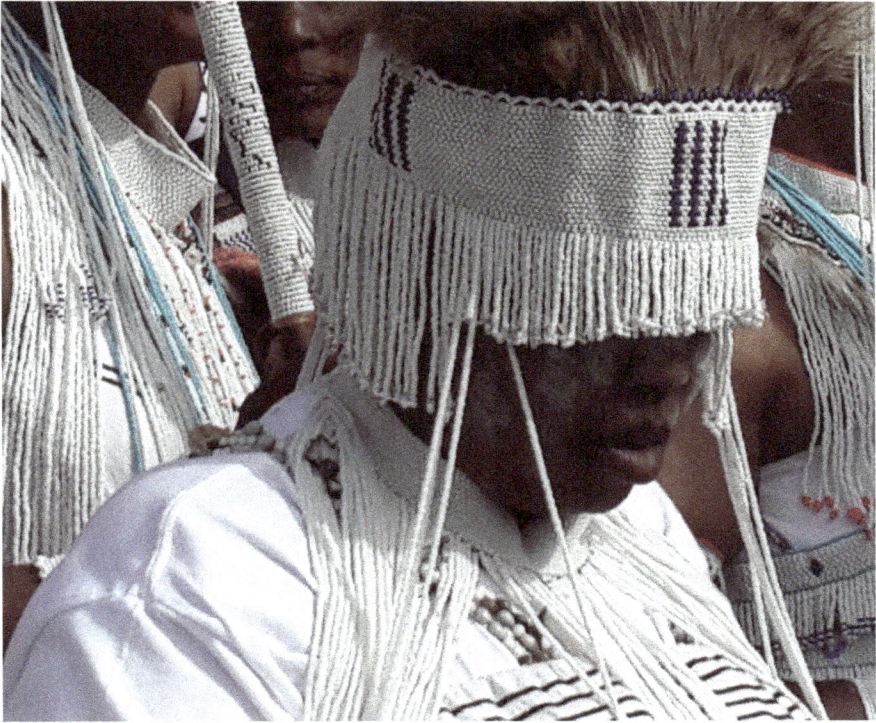

Figure 26: An initiate displays the head piece with the white beads

In the analytical realm, the idea of dismemberment can apply to the breaking down of one-sided ego attitudes that no longer serve the personality and to the differentiation of archetypal dream images into smaller, more understandable parts so that their meaning can be digested or assimilated into consciousness. Within the African healing paradigm, this theme is further symbolized by the ritual sacrifices at each stage of the initiation.

Animal Sacrifice and Initiation

The idea of animal sacrifice is an anathema to the Western mind. It is a phenomenon that is the root of many misperceptions and the vilification of this belief system. It remains a phenomenon that continues to challenge my own relationship with animals and my Western-based ideas. As such, I have been motivated to try to understand the symbolic aspect embedded in these rituals. For the healer, these sacrifices are carefully constructed to forge a link between the human initiate and the ancestors. The ritual of the animal sacrifice is found in most indigenous practices and is archetypal in nature. Psychologically, the ritual embodies the drive or instinct to establish a connection between the ego and the Self.

Edinger (1972) enumerated the features of the archetypal sacrificial ritual to include an unblemished animal, a ritualized sacrificial killing, a blood libation to gods, and the dividing of the flesh between man and god in which the human portion is consumed and the god portion burned. The animal sacrifice can be understood as the ego's willingness to sacrifice the instinctual urges, thereby gaining some control over these urges and in turn participating in the transformation and humanization of the God-image. Thus the symbolic meaning of the sacrifice, as explained by Edinger (1972), is a necessary act performed by man in order to nourish the gods. That is, psychologically, the ego supports the self-movement from the human to the divine. Jung (1954c) noted that:

> What is performed concretely on the sacrificial animal, and what the shaman believes to be actually happening to himself, appears on a higher level . . . as a psychic process in which a product of the unconscious . . . is cut up and transformed. . . . He is essentially unconscious and therefore in need of transformation and enlightenment. For this purpose his body must be taken apart and dissolved into its constituents, a process known in alchemy as the division, *separatio* and *solutio*, discrimination and self-knowledge. (para. 411)

Animal sacrifice can be understood psychologically as instinctual energy, which must be extracted from the unconscious. Through the sacrificial act, one experiences a conscious encounter with primitive instinctive drives in the faith that they are capable of being transformed. The main purpose of the sacrifice here is to ensure the presence and participation of the ancestors (see Radomsky, 2017). This is, in part, achieved via the incorporation of parts of the animal in the initiate's regalia and ritualized eating of the sacrifice. Jung (1952b) commented on the numinosity of the sacrifice, and he observed that:

The animal-sacrifice, where it has lost its original meaning as an offered gift and has taken on a higher religious significance, has an inner relationship to the hero or god. The animal represents the god himself; thus the bull represents Dionysus . . . the lamb, Christ. (para. 659)

The three predominant sacrificial animals within this healing realm, which are central to the initiation of the healers, are the chicken, the goat, and the cow or bull (see Ntombi's initial dream in chapter 5). All the animals are carefully selected, are required to be blemish free, and are usually seen in a dream by the initiate to indicate the readiness to progress further.

Each animal sacrifice is considered sacred and auspicious. The animals are carefully prepared, and after the sacrifice, no part of the animal is wasted. The skins are seen as a direct gift from the ancestors, and the initiate is expected to keep the skin as part of the regalia and for the making of the drums. The gallbladder is removed, as are the vertebrae. These are treated with oils and are woven into the regalia of the initiate. The meat is roasted, part of which is given to the ancestors and part of which is eaten by the initiate and healers. The offer to the ancestors is left in the ancestor's position in the hut. The ritual surrounding the animal sacrifice is formal and symbolic. The initiate and healers partake of the sacrificial meats while ensuring that a portion is left for the ancestors.

An amplification of the Promethean myth wherein Prometheus presided over the procedure of dividing the meat of the sacrifices between gods and men, suggests the archetypal aspect of the sacrifice. The process of dividing the meat of the sacrificial animal represents a separation of the ego from the archetypal psyche or self. The ego, as Edinger (1972) explained, in order to establish itself as an autonomous entity, must appropriate the food or energy for itself (p. 24). Within the African healing cosmology, the animal sacrifice heralds the initiate's separation from the collective community and the beginning of the individual journey to becoming the healer.

The numinosity of the sacrifice is highlighted in the amplification of the archetypal patterns underlying these rituals. The sacrificial rituals unfold in relation to differing numerical rhythms and correspond to the increasing proficiency of the initiate, psychologically, to a development in consciousness.

Number Symbolism and the Stages of the Sacrifice

Each ceremony, which includes a sacrifice, unfolds over a different number of days (see also Radomsky, 2017). Von Franz, in her book *Number and Time* (1974), offered a unique, complex, and in-depth account of the relationship between number symbolism and the objective psyche. The relevant focus for this work is predominantly the qualitative aspect of number in contradistinction to the occidental quantitative aspect (see von Franz, *Number and Time*, 1974, for a full explanation). In applying the concept of natural numbers to the rhythms embedded in the rituals, the idea of a qualitative aspect of numbers becomes immediately apparent.

The main idea here is to highlight the symbolic nature of numbers as images of the archetype of order (Jung, 1952c, para. 870) and the nature of number as a continuous rather than a discontinuous concept wherein each number qualitatively contains an indivisible whole. Von Franz (1974) elaborates: "The concept of natural numbers rests on an archetypal foundation. It represents a preconscious pattern of thought common to all human psyches, and therefore constitutes the basis for transmitting knowledge" (p. 301). It is this characteristic of number that seems useful in amplifying the stages of the initiation ritual, as each stage is in and of itself a completion of an aspect of the individuation process. To quote von Franz (1974):

> Numbers then become typical psychological patterns of motion about which we can make the following statements: One comprises wholeness, two divides, repeats, and engenders symmetries, three centers the symmetries and initiates successions, four acts as a stabilizer by turning back to the one ... each number, taken qualitatively, is understood to function as a preconscious psychic principle of activity; each number must be thought of as containing a specific activity that ... signify different rhythmic configurations of the one-continuum. (p. 74-75)

Von Franz further explained the idea that the patterns underlying this preconscious aspect of natural numbers hint at a "numerical *field*" in which the individual numbers carry a certain energetic influence or "rhythmical configuration" (1974, p. 303). By "field," von Franz was hinting at the collective unconscious and the archetype of the Self. Here she emphasized that the characteristics of the natural numbers "appear to constitute the most basic constants of nature expressing unitary psychophysical reality" (1974, p. 303). Von Franz was referring to Jung's idea that numbers are not merely conscious constructs, but are aspects of nature:

> Numbers appear to represent both an attribute of matter and the unconscious foundation of our mental processes . . . numbers form that particular element that unites the realms of matter and psyche. It is "real" in a double sense, as an archetypal image and as a qualitative manifestation in the realm of outer-world experience. (1974, p. 52)

Jung further suggested that the archetypes of natural numbers might be linked with the concept of the *unus mundus*, the one world and the collective unconscious. It is this idea that, for me, seems to underlie the structures embedded in the initiatory ceremonies of the animal sacrifice.

To be clear, my idea here emerged from my observations of the initiatory rituals. The ceremonies for each of the sacrificial stages seem to embody an informal inherent pattern, reflected, in part, in the number of days for each ritual. The neophyte, in an initial state of unconsciousness, shifts toward a differentiated consciousness as the fully fledged healer, in touch with the realm of the transpersonal unity that underlies psyche and matter—the *unus mundus*.

Each sacrifice marks the level of this transformation in the proficiency of the initiate. As such, the amplification of the numbers with respect to each of the initiatory stages seems to offer us yet another image of Jung's hypothesis, as elaborated by von Franz (1992), that "number is a quantity *and* an active specific qualitative manifestation of the one-continuum, i.e., the *unus mundus*" (p. 54).

The Chicken Sacrifice

The whitening stage of the *ukuthwasa* initiation begins with the sacrifice of the white chicken. This sacrifice is the inauguration ritual of the *albedo* stage, performed to inform the ancestors that a new initiate has answered the calling and is preparing for the training. The chicken is carefully selected to be blemish free and completely white. Chickens in everyday life are usually associated with cowardice and stupidity; symbolically they are also related to gold via the color of their feet. Legend has it that they stirred the molten gold with their feet and absorbed it completely (de Vries, 1974). In this way, the chicken carries that which is of the highest value as well as a capacity to heal, as seen in the colloquial making of chicken broth for ailments. Both these qualities are needed by the dreamer in order for her to embrace her calling as healer.

The chicken can be amplified as a symbol of fertility and devoted motherhood (mother hen). The scratching motion of the feet that is so characteristic of the chicken is thought to have brought the world into being. An important amplification for our purposes is the feature of the hen brooding over her eggs. A sitting hen suggests a psychic brooding essential to the process of transformation and evokes within the African cosmology the brooding of the ancestors that are said to hover over and sit on the neophyte until something transforms. The chicken is also associated with rebirth through the egg, which is a primordial symbol of the Self. Jung (1955–56) cites the alchemist John Dee, who speculates that "the center of nature is 'the point originated by God,' the 'sun-point' in the egg" (para. 41). This central core of the egg, the yolk or the "chick-point," is the mystic germ brooded into life by the heat of the hen, symbolic of the heat of the unconscious, akin to the meditation of the adept.

This ritual serves to release the initiate from the tortuous darkness of the *nigredo*. At this time, there was a noticeable shift in Ntombi's depressive symptoms and she described a feeling of immense relief and liberation. In Alchemy, the release from earthly constraints of the *nigredo* through the operation of the *sublimatio* is often symbolized by the white bird flying up out of matter or the extraction of spirit from matter (see Edinger, 1991, p. 121).

The Chicken and the Number One

The ceremony in which the chicken sacrifice is central usually takes place over one day and is a communal ritual. The amplification of the number symbolism is relevant here as the creative aspect of the number reflects the dynamic as well as the archetypal character of the rituals. The number one stands before the beginning of all ordering, before the creative process begins (Apt, 2005). One is the individual number and the basis of all natural numbers, and it is a symbol for the still undivided wholeness, the origin, a primal unconsciousness before differentiation. Von Franz (1974) elaborated that the one is also symbolic of the result of the creative process, the end point or goal of individuation, symbolizing the final union of everything and linked to the supreme Godhead. The one characterizes an archaic identity and consciously a sense of oneness with all creation.

The single day in which the initial sacrifice occurs evokes images of the creation, as in Genesis: "and there was evening and there was morning, one day" (1:5). This refers to the beginning of differentiation between the light and the dark out of the initial chaos or *prima materia*. Jung (1955–56) reflected on the one day in this way and further refers to the symbolism of Mercurius, named the "son of one day" and a symbol of the light of the first day of creation (para. 476, 718). Thus, in the one day we have the symbolism of a beginning as well as a totality or *coniunctio*, as Mercurius, as a symbol

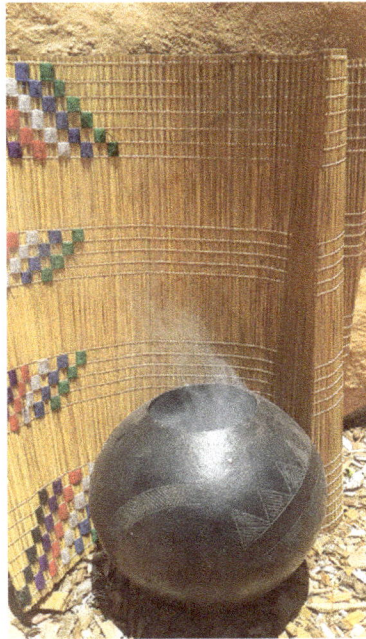

Figure 27. The burning of white *muthi*

of the outcome of the alchemical opus, embodies a union of opposites. The symbolism of the one includes a return to the one as a transformed totality, at the end of the process. The ultimate aim of the creative process, according to von Franz (1974), is a return to an undivided wholeness, with consciousness. This is captured in alchemical axiom of Maria Prophetissa: "Out of the One comes Two, out of Two comes Three, and from the Third comes the One as the Fourth" (quoted in von Franz 1974, p. 65). It is significant therefore, that this initial ceremony takes place over one day where the neophyte, in an undifferentiated and unconscious state, begins a journey toward differentiation, the development of healing capacities, and autonomy.

The whitening phase is further characterized by the use of the *imithi emhlope* (white medicines) representing ultimate well-being, and the effect of this *muthi* is to open the dream pathways and clear communications with the ancestors. The Zulu word for this phenomenon is *ubulawu*, which means "to open the mind to dreams and to the messages from the ancestors."

These white herbs are either vaporized or distilled and ingested during the initial *albedo* stage of the initiation. For African healers, the white *muthi* is the feminine cleansing milk that both nourishes and sustains the acolyte on her journey. This *muthi* is used to awaken intuition and the lunar energies, a symbolic ascent to heavenly realms. This will be followed by the reddening and a return to earthly embodiment.

Chapter 7
Imithi Ebomuvu:
The Red Medicine

The ancestor's voice comes into you.
This is the time to hand over the energy.
—Ntombi

The next stage of the *ukuthwasa* initiation, akin to the alchemical *rubedo,* is marked by the introduction of the color red, the end of the period of celibacy, and the goat sacrifice. The outer apparel of the initiate is changed from white to red cloth, accompanied by red beads, and the body and face are painted with red clay. This stage heralds the shift from the introverted and more spiritualized aspect of the whitening or *albedo*, to a more embodied materialized awareness or consciousness.

As Ntombi entered this stage of the initiatory process, her doubts about the authenticity of her calling returned. Once more she found herself engulfed in the darkness of her depression. Her therapeutic process was a complex one, marked by suicidal ideations, often when the dreams would not simply "go away." She felt I had failed her in that I had not taken on her projection of the white goddess who would magically extract her from her cultural matrix and stop the emergence of unconscious material.

Once again, the opposites were reflected in our process and a new understanding emerged for me. I became alert to the transforming potential of otherness in the relationship. My awareness extended to the possibility of being overcome with the immensity of the responsibility of these numinous experiences, or falling into inflation, if this experience was not tempered by the sense of something in the background, something beyond the personal, the awareness of the Self that supported and guided the process. I was cognizant of the need to hold Ntombi's projection in the transference, which was at times intense and almost too hot to bear.

This intensity required a careful awareness of whether or not there was a risk of melting in the fire of the unconscious or whether the fiery heat would be transformative and something would endure, often symbolized in alchemy by the salamander able to withstand the heat of the fire. My own dreams at this time seemed to offer support and encouragement. I dreamed:

I am with three healers, two men and a woman. They invite me to enter an underground cavern. In the centre of the cavern is a natural pool of water. The water glows with a deep crimson. The healers explain that the color is a reflection of the red crystal stone matrix of the cave. A voice says "this is the pool of life."

It was in the holding of that elusive threshold between opposites that an alchemical process seemed to be at work. It was only due to my own experiences in the initiatory realm that this was, in any way, possible. Ntombi shared the following dream as a compensation for her one-sided conscious standpoint:

I'm lying in my bed. I wake up (in the dream) to see my grandfather standing over me. He was very old, older than he was when he died. He's standing over me and he is holding a baby. I say "what a beautiful baby." He says, "Well, it is yours and I would not like to see this baby dirty or hungry. So look after this child. Wake up and go and tell your father that it is time I rested. So go and take the goat and do the ritual so that I can rest."

Ntombi expressed feeling calm and peaceful after this dream. The dream seemed to shift her acceptance of her calling to the point where her fear was no longer so palpable. This acceptance was encouraged by another numinous dream image. She dreamed:

I am walking under the water in the ocean. In front of me is a row of candles, alight in the water. I follow the candles and arrive at the other side. On the shore, three goats are standing. A voice says these are the goats for your sacrifice. When I woke, I knew that I was ready for the next stage. I would have to sacrifice three goats.

The image of the candles alight despite being under the water seemed to offer Ntombi confirmation of a connection to something otherworldly and mysterious. She commented that she felt that she was on the right path, and she could see her way forward. Here the dream seems to offer another image of the *ortus solis* or an illumination after the darkness.

The Dawning of Consciousness

The alchemical *citrinitas* is, at times, an intermediary stage during the transition from the whitening to the reddening. Jung (1955–56) mentioned the "four-footed '*Ortus*,' which combines in itself the four alchemical colors, black, red, white and yellow" (para. 281). In *Psychology and Alchemy* (1944) Jung referred to the yellow of the *citrinitas* as corresponding to the red of the *rubedo*. However, in many alchemical writings, this stage is often overlooked or considered less significant. For example, Marie-Louise von Franz, in her text *Alchemy* (1980a), does not mention the *citrinitas*. In a later text, von Franz (1998) collates the stage of the *rubedo* with the *citrinitas*. Jung commented that the stage of the *citrinitas* seemed to belong to an earlier formulation of the alchemical process, which later fell into disuse. Jung carries on with the idea that the four stages signified a quaternity and this seemed to evolve into three, a trinity, most likely due to inner psychological reasons at the time.

Similarly, the uncertainty of the position of yellowing is reflected in the *ukuthwasa* process. There is no formal identifiable sacrifice to mark a transition from the whitening to a yellowing before the reddening. However, observing and participating in many initiations across different tribes, I came across a yellowing phase in a few instances where the initiate was deemed to be in an emerging state between the white and the red. In these cases, the change in status was marked exclusively by the addition of yellow cloth to the initiate's white regalia. The yellowing, in the African healing worldview (and in the alchemical opus) seems to indicate the beginning of the emergence of consciousness, or the realization that the contents of the unconscious have an actualized reality. For the initiate this would mean the emerging relationship with the ancestors and the initiate's readiness to begin the next stage of the reddening.

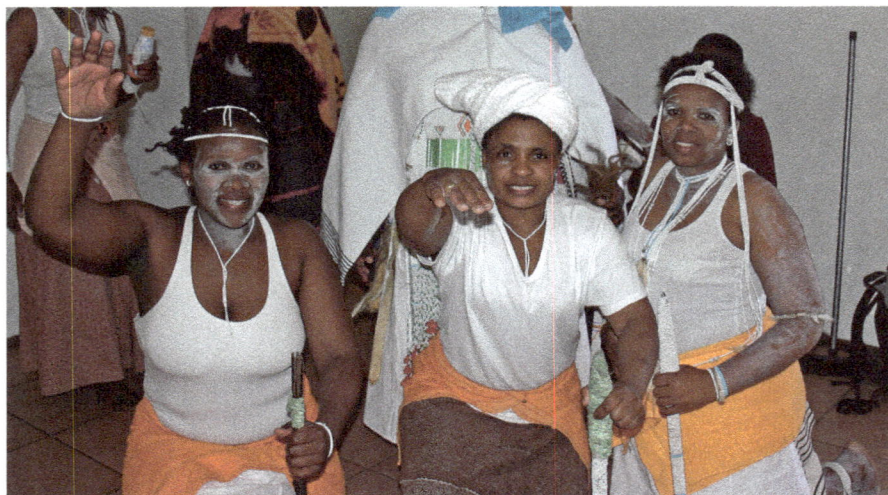

Figure 28. Three initiates still with the white of the *albedo* phase,
but with the addition of yellow cloth tied around their waists

The reddening heralds the initiate's seniority. It is the stage just prior to the culmination of the initiation. The time of inner preparation of the whitening stage is over, and the initiate now begins to activate the healing powers and skills cultivated in the previous stage. The *thwasa* becomes active in the healing rituals, assisting the senior healers and participating in the cultivation and distillation of the herbal remedies. Under the guidance of the experienced healers, the *thwasa* begins to diagnose illnesses, and the channel to the ancestral communications is deemed to be open and accessible. Von Franz (1998) clarifies that the *rubedo* essentially marks the end of the hard work where "the retort is opened and the philosophers' stone begins to radiate a cosmically healing effect" (p. 227).

The inclusion of the red color signifies coming alive—psychologically, an animation of consciousness—and the birth of the mature healer, now able to function more independently. Red embodies the vivifying, enlivening, and renewing energy but can be a dangerous time, as the red hot fiery heat that can also burn. The healers comment that the transition to this stage is only possible if the initiate has traversed the previous stage successfully in that there is the development of a humble attitude in the face of ancestral energies. In other words, if the initiate is aware of her conscious position relative to the inner authority of the psyche, this guards against inflations or the potentially dangerous heat of the fire.

The Goat Sacrifice

The culmination of the red stage is marked by the ritual sacrifice of the goat. In Africa, the goat embodies both procreative and protective powers, and the wearing of a goatskin was said to bring one closer to the ancestors. The goat is a paradoxical symbol that embodies both the dark and the light. The goat is associated with fertility as well as licentiousness, evoking images of Pan and the devil. Von Franz (1980a) observed that the blood of the goat is said to have corrosive qualities that can destroy everything. Goat's blood was also said to possess extraordinary powers and to absorb disease, and goats were often the guardians of medieval villages. These amplifications are relevant here as the goat sacrifice heralds the end to the period of celibacy and an intermediary stage in the development of the autonomy of the initiate who is now deemed able to perform healing rituals under supervision of an experienced healer.

During the goat ceremony, blood forms a central part of the sacrificial ritual. The blood of the animal is collected and mixed with healing herbs. The amplification of the blood symbolism reveals that blood is often the *prima materia*. As Jung (1944) expanded: "The basis of the opus, the *prima materia* . . . represents the unknown substance that carries the projection of the autonomous psychic content" (para. 425). The *prima materia* took different forms for the individual alchemists, which included mercurial quicksilver, water, gold, fire, earth, and blood, among many other substances. Throughout mythology, blood forms an integral part of rituals and ceremonies, evoking both power and fear, and symbolically suggesting the seat of life or the soul. In many indigenous systems the shades or ancestors could be restored to life by drinking blood. Blood is the essence of life itself, carries suprapersonal connotations, and was thought to belong to the gods. It is the blood that forms the covenant between man and god (Exodus 24:4–8). Thus the most appropriate gift to the gods is the blood sacrifice. The priestesses of Apollo drank the blood of the sacrificial lamb in order to commune with the gods and to prophesy. The Masai of Kenya drink the blood of animals in order to bond with the animals' nature. Blood is seen as the divine fluid and thought to be autonomous and able to act of its own accord. Edinger (1995) reflects on the symbolic power of blood to attract the spirits of the dead, in that "the unconscious is brought into connection with consciousness by the sacrifice of blood" (p. 294).

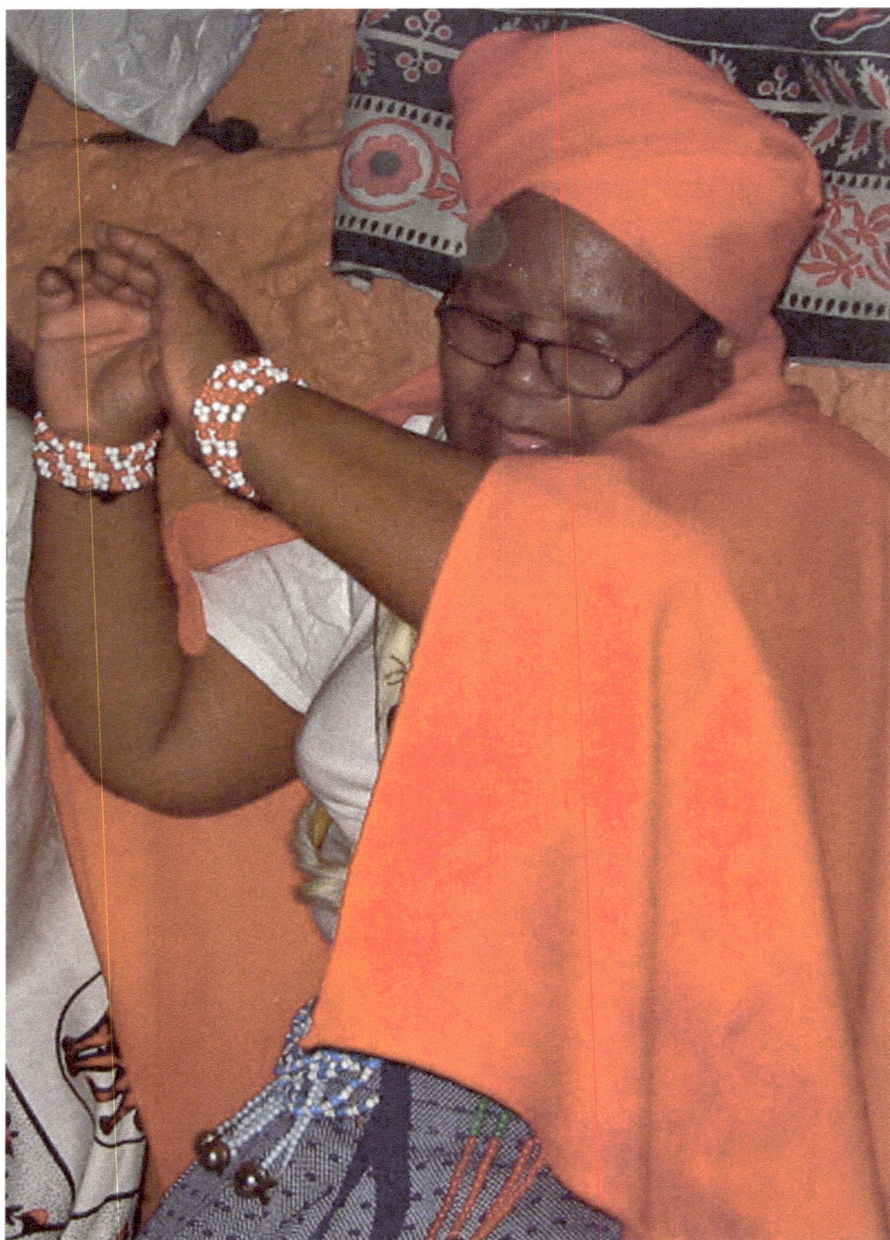

Figure 29. A healer during the reddening phase wearing
the red head piece and shawl of the regalia

After the spiritualization of the *albedo* phase, the *rubedo* is characterized by the soul's return to the body and the exaltation of matter. In the transformation from the *albedo* to the *rubedo,* the symbolism of the blood is essential. As Jung (1977) commented, "blood alone can re-animate a glorious state of consciousness in which the last trace of blackness is dissolved" (p. 229).

The Goat and the Number Three

The goat ceremony often unfolds over three days, including the preparations for the ceremony, the selection of the appropriate animal and the actual day of the sacrifice.[15] It is interesting to recall that in Ntombi's dream three goats appeared. In most instances, the initiate is only required to sacrifice one goat in this ceremony. However, in honoring the ancestral wishes in her dream, Ntombi was required to select three goats for her sacrifice. After the sacrifice Ntombi dreamed that the three goats returned to her in the form of ancestral spirits.

Three indicates dynamism and change, the emergence of something new and an irreversible process in time. Time is experienced as a trinity of past, present, and future, and three is the fateful aspect that develops out of two. Jung (2008) explained that "the Three stands in connection to time. The Three is time, and time is always identical with the *flow of energy* (p. 204).

Von Franz (1974) reminds us that the number three, the triadic structure, appears frequently in myths and fairy tales. It takes the form of three tasks that the hero must perform before the final transformation. There are often three questions that must be asked of the oracle in order to gain entry beyond a certain threshold. This is also a precarious stage in the emergence of the creative transformation in that unconscious content potentially crosses the threshold of consciousness. Von Franz (1992) cautions that the "three . . . symbolizes that that very archetype is actively possessing the ego, forcing upon it actions or thoughts" (p. 283).

The three days and completion of the goat ceremony mark the beginning of the initiate's separation from the dependence on the mentor. With the successful culmination of the goat ceremony, the initiate emerges as an apprentice healer recognized as having attained the healing ability.

Here the qualitative symbolism of the three seems applicable. As Jung (1948c) indicated:

> Every tension of opposites culminates in a release, out of which comes the "third." In the third, the tension is resolved and the lost unity restored. Unity, the absolute One, cannot be numbered, it is indefinable and unknowable; only when it appears as a unit, the number one, is it knowable, for the "Other" which is required for this act of knowing is lacking in the condition of the One. Three is the unfolding of the One to a condition where it can be known. (para. 180)

Thus the three possesses a knowable quality, beyond the unknowable unity of the one and the oscillatory tension of the two from which the three is "birthed." In other words, as von Franz (1974) explained: "Threefold rhythms are most probably connected with processes in space and time or with their realization in consciousness" (p. 109). Triadic structures further appear in the oracle of the *I Ching*, as well as in genetic research into the structures of DNA and RNA. Once again, von Franz (1974) elucidates when she asserts that:

> One cannot escape the impression that these numerical combinations are introspective representations of fundamental processes in our psychological nature. . . . The messenger RNA . . . uses triplets to form the basic figures of its code. In these genetic findings we are confronted with an exchange of "information" in living cells that corresponds exactly to the structure of the I Ching hexagrams. (p. 106)

This correspondence seems to support Jung's hypothesis that "the individual aspect of number appears to contain the mysterious factor that enables it to organize psyche and matter jointly" (von Franz, 1974, p. 61). As von Franz (1974) clearly explains: "Three signifies a unity which dynamically engenders self-expanding linear irreversible processes in matter and in our consciousness" (p. 106). Three, psychologically, is that which emerges from the tension of the two, which we can understand as a birth of consciousness. Thus three suggests "a development toward a personal standpoint, a new insight or new symbol, the beginning of a new, fateful development" (Apt, 2005, p. 124).

After the goat sacrifice, the apprentice healer undergoes ongoing training and refinement of skills that can continue for a number of years. This is the stage when the channel of communication with the ancestors is honed and perfected. At this stage the initiate begins to demonstrate an increased capacity for healing. Psychologically, the initiate develops a relationship with the unconscious and learns to trust in the autonomy of the objective psyche.

The Alchemical *Coagulatio*

The initiate's developing autonomy is akin to the alchemical operation of the *coagulatio*, which is the process of solidifying, returning to earth and the reemergence of libidinal energies. After the spiritualization of the whitening, something concrete must incarnate in the *thwasa* in order for the full healing capacity to be realized. As Edinger (1972) pointed out, this is the process of psychic development where the ego emerges from a state of oneness with the objective psyche, a state that is experienced during the initial stage of the *ukuthwasa* initiation.

Following the severe restrictions and rituals of the whitening during which ego desires are sublimated and spiritualized, the transition to the reddening is the return to ego consciousness and the coagulation of the archetypal and numinous experiences into the healing ability of the mature healer. Edinger (1991) explained that "the *coagulatio* . . . expresses the archetypal process of ego formation. . . . When the ego's relation to the Self is being realized" (p. 115). The red phase of *ukuthwasa* initiation is marked by an experience that the healers describe as "being gripped by something." This is comparable to von Franz's (1980a) description of the *rubedo* in analysis in that it should release us from the experience that grips or falls upon us as from above, resulting in "an experience that has substance and body" (p. 296).

From a psychological perspective, psychic contents are said to be brought to earth or to become embodied. That is, following the submersion in the *albedo*, a return to matter is necessary. As noted by Edward Edinger

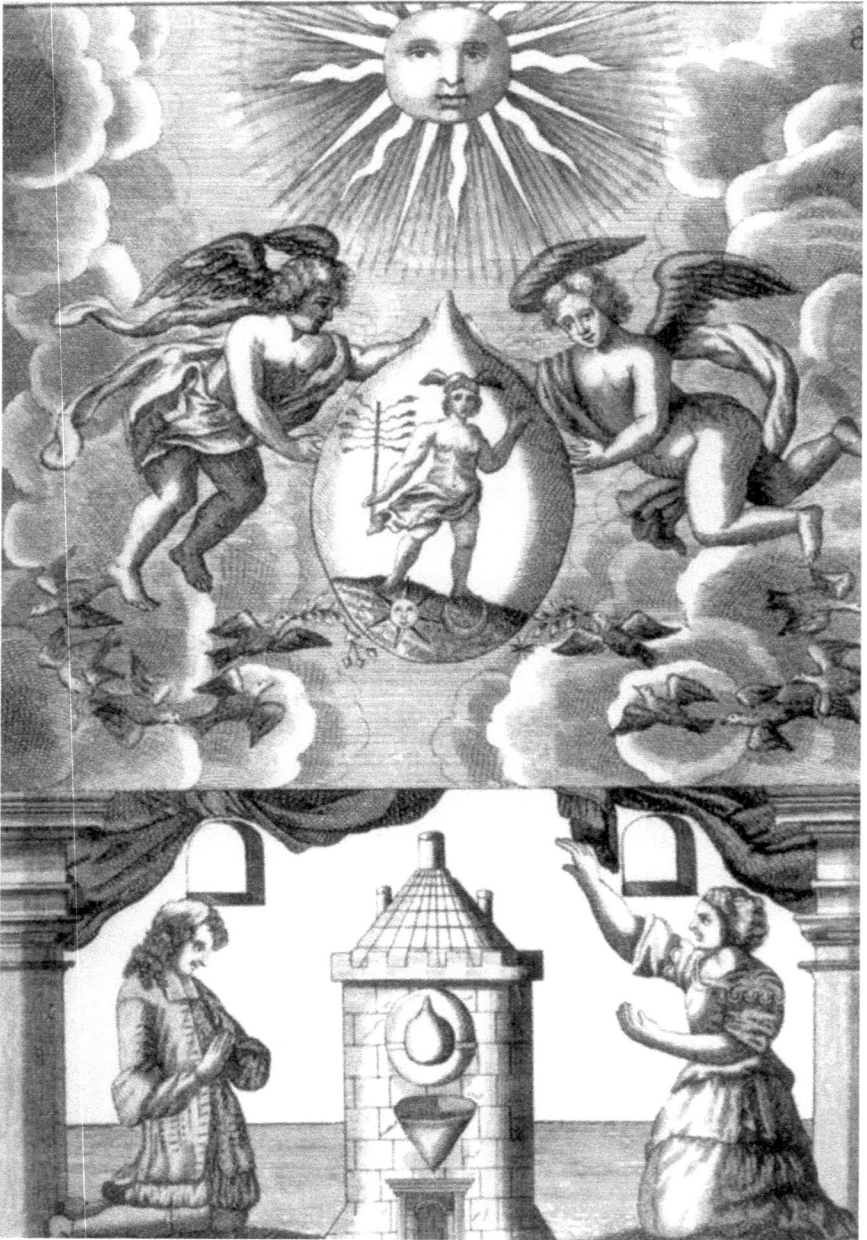

Figure 30. The upper two thirds show Mecurius in the "philosopher's egg" or the alchemical vessel. The heat of the sun, symbolic of consciousness, warms the vessel from above as the furnace does from below. The lower third depicts two alchemists at work, kneeling before the furnace below symbolizing the unconscious *Mutus liber* Plate 8

(1991), the *coagulatio* is the operation of relationship wherein something coagulates and solidifies, where spirit materializes in matter.

For the alchemist, this spirit is an aspect of the spirit Mercurius, psychologically, the paradoxical nature of the autonomous psyche.[16] For the individual, this is similar to the mercurial nature of the experience of being gripped by a complex. The assimilation and the integration of such a complex—becoming conscious of the effect of the complex—is akin to a *coagulatio*.

For Ntombi, this, in part, meant the confrontation with her "need to be white" complex and the resultant emerging capacity to embrace a more authentic ego identity. At this time, a dream arrives that seems to suggest the transformation occurring for Ntombi. She dreamed:

> *I'm walking deep in the forest. There is an older woman with me, a healer. We arrive in the centre of the forest where there is a huge old tree. I cannot see the top it's so tall and the branches extend out seemingly forever. The tree seems to be completely engulfed by flames and yet is not being destroyed by the fire. I notice one branch that seems different from the others. I reach up to grab it and as I pull it, a door opened in the tree trunk – a small opening. I reach inside and lying deep in the tree is a crystal that seems to glow with a red light and fits perfectly in my hand. The woman tells me that the crystal must become a part of my healing tools.*

The symbols in the dream of the tree, the fire that does not burn and the red crystal seemed to confirm Ntombi's evolution on her path of becoming the healer. The tree encompasses one of the most profound, multi-layered and ubiquitous symbols found in almost all cultural, mythological, spiritual, and religious traditions. The image of the tree symbolizes the link between the transcendent heavens and earthly domain, and epitomizes the image of the archetype of eternal life and regeneration. In reaching upwards into the heavens and downwards into the underworld, the tree is a symbol of the cosmos, transcending space and time.

The universality of the tree symbol in which is embodied its pre-destined nature, rooted deep in the universe, psychologically has come to represent an image of the process of achieving consciousness, or the individuation process rooted deep in the Self. On an individual level, for

Ntombi, the symbol of the tree in the context of the dream evokes a multigenerational image, akin to the family tree, the lineage of her family tradition.

For the alchemists the tree is a central symbol of the opus, a symbol of the *prima materia* and the union of opposites, which depicts the nature of inner life, a place of awakening, but also the place of death, suffering and sacrifice. In many indigenous rituals, the tree represents the umbilicus to the underworld, the birth canal as well as a conduit for the communication with the gods (compare to the burning bush at which Moses is instructed by the voice of God in Exodus 3:1-4:17). As Jung (1938) expands:

> In the history of symbols, this tree is described as the way of life itself, a growing into that which eternally is and does not change; which springs from the union of opposites and, by its eternal presence, also makes that union possible. It seems as if it were only through an experience of symbolic reality that man, vainly seeking his own "existence" and making a philosophy out of it, can find his way back to a world in which he is no longer a stranger (para. 198).

The Alchemical *Calcinatio*

In the *ukuthwasa* initiation, burning is central at this reddening stage and is related to the alchemical operation of *calcinatio*. Healers are said to be unaffected by the destructive heat of the fire, symbolized in the dream by the tree that does not burn. At this stage in the initiation the initiates are required to pick up burning coals or take a burning pot off the fire with their mouths and to demonstrate that they have not been burned. This signifies the protective spirit of the ancestors, who render the initiates immune to the fire. This phenomenon is well documented across a number of indigenous and shamanistic initiations, including those found in India, Tibet, China, and Japan and in the Native American cultures in South and North America. Edinger (1991) noted that the "image of invulnerability to fire indicates an immunity to identification with affect" (p. 24).

Psychologically, we can understand this symbolism as the ego consciousness having been matured and humbled through the contact with the objective psyche to the level of being less identified with affective heat of the fiery emotions or less identified with the autonomous unconscious content. At this stage, the heat of the fire has both a purifying as well as solidifying effect.

Edinger (1991) explains that the heat of the fire "alludes to the integration of the personality through the process of *calcinatio*" (p. 30). This is an outcome of the initiation wherein the initiate has developed into a mature healer able to withstand the effects of the libidinal fire both internally and externally.

Within most indigenous systems, fire and sacrifice to the gods are connected. Fire was thought of as the connecting link between the human and the divine realms. Edinger (1991) explained that what was burned in the sacrifice was made sacred and became numinous, linking the human to the divine through the ascent of the smoke, an image of matter becoming spirit (p. 38). He quotes the Syrian philosopher Iamblichus, who notes that in the Greek *thysia*, or sacrificial rite,

> the energy of divine fire destroys everything which is material in sacrifices, purifies things which are offered, liberates them from the bonds of matter, renders them through the purity of nature . . . to the communication of the gods . . . and conducts our material nature to an immaterial essence. (1991, p. 40)

According to Jung (1997a), if one is governed by ego desires, one is possessed, but if one is conscious of these desires, they

> slowly get quiet and transform, and you will discern that in the bottle grows a stone . . . in as much as self-control . . . has become a habit, it is a stone . . . when it has become a *fait accompli*, it is a diamond. (p. 614)

The crystal in Ntombi's dream, like the stone, is a symbol of the Self (see chapter 2). Jung (1944) described the alchemical Hermetic vessel, the "*vas Hermetis*," which contained the substances to be transformed, "a kind of matrix or uterus from which the *filius philosophorum*, the miraculous stone, is . . . born" (para. 338). For the initiate, the *vas* is the healer-novice relationship, akin to the analytical relationship. It is in the temenos of the therapeutic relationship that transformation occurs. Psychologically, this transformation will require a certain strengthening of the ego in relation to the numinosity of the Self. As Edinger (1991) elucidated:

> The fire of the *calcinatio*, to the extent that it can be brought about by the psychotherapist, is achieved largely by expressing attitudes and reactions that frustrate the patient. . . . A sufficiently solid psychic foundation must be present to endure the *calcinatio*, and also an adequate rapport between the patient and the therapist must exist to be able to carry the frustration without generating destructive negativity. (p. 43)

At this stage of the initiation, fire symbolism is at its most prominent in an aspect of this ceremony called the "burning of the bones." The bones of the sacrificial animal, as well as all the regalia worn by the initiate during the previous stages of the initiation, are burned, signifying both a final transformation and coming together of all the levels achieved along with the purification of all previous stages of the personality. The fire ceremony amplified as the *calcinatio* symbolizes an integration of the personality of the mature healer. This is revisited at the end of the initiation process with the graduation of the fully evolved healer (see chapter 8).

This ceremony seems to evoke a further form of purification. After the *calcinatio*, ashes remain, in which are contained the supreme value or goal of the work, as the ash is the incorruptible glorified body that has survived the purifying fire, a new psychic substance. The purification effect of the fires relates psychologically to the drying out of the unconscious affects, the transformation of desirousness, and the power drive. As von Franz (1980a) described, the burning of the *prima materia* ensures that all destructive humidity has been removed and all that is left are the ashes, the driest substance (p. 228). By treating the *prima materia* with fire or water, the alchemists intended to extract the divine creative power of spirit from the darkness of matter. We can think of the *Śarīra*, the crystal beads purportedly found in the cremated ashes of Buddhist spiritual masters.

Psychologically, the burning is the removing of different kinds of unconsciousness, blind spots, unconscious assumptions, and projections, which are obstacles to development and corrupt our perceptions. It seems appropriate that at the point just before the initiate potentially graduates as a mature healer, there is a final burning away and refining of ego-driven desires, unconscious complexes and contaminations.

Ntombi reported a dream during this phase in which her own body had to be burned to ashes during the sacrifice. Her ashes were then collected in a bottle and mixed with blood and regenerated. Here we are reminded of the nourishing living waters or the natural humidity about which the alchemists spoke. From a psychological standpoint, the recollection of corruptible projections and unconsciousness is often brings relief and the clarity of the pure living waters. Things can be seen for what they are.

For the mature healer, this final burning of the bones, symbolizes the transformation of ego desires and pursuits into healing abilities. This is essential if the healer is to function from an authentic position without identification with the healer archetype. The ashes from the burning ceremony are buried at the doorway to the healer's hut, which is also the seat of the ancestors, symbolizing once again a *coniunctio* of spirit and matter.

During this stage red herbs are prepared, the *imithi ebomuvu* (red medicines). These are the protective and strengthening medicines as the healers consider this stage the most difficult and important of the entire initiation process. The initiation culminates in the final sacrifice of the cow or the bull. This final ceremony heralds the incarnation of the umbilicus between healer and the ancestors.

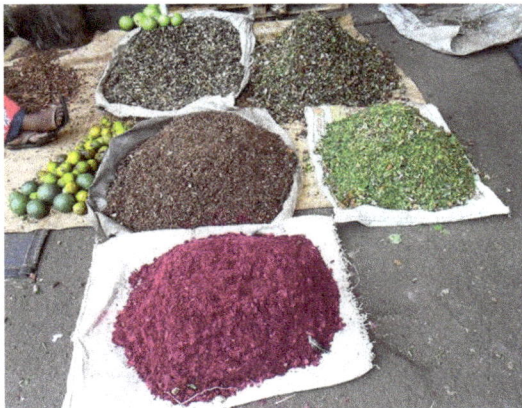

Figure 31. Herbs at *muthi* market with the red herbs in the front

Chapter 8
Ukuphothula:
The Final Awakening

Deep down, I knew that this is who I am.
I answered the ancestral way.
—Ntombi

A central outcome of the *ukuthwasa* initiation, from a psychological understanding, is the evolution of the inner dialectic between the ego and the
Self. The initiation rituals serve the purpose of strengthening ego consciousness in order to withstand the development of an inner gradient toward the
Self. Ntombi's progress was validated in the following numinous dream:

> *I am asleep in my grandfather's kraal. Something wakes me and I
> notice a white light outside the entryway. Two African men and a
> woman enter. The woman leads in a cow. The cow is magnificent,
> black and white and on her head, between her huge crescent-
> shaped horns, is a golden disk.*

Ntombi responded with a sense of awe about the dream. She
recognized that this dream, relative to her cultural understanding, was a
final verification of her calling. Dreams, which had been central throughout
the initiation, become even more pivotal at this time. The *thwasa* cannot
proceed with the ultimate phase of the initiation until a dream appears
indicating the readiness for this level of transformation. Such a dream will
also decide whether the sacrificial animal for the last ritual will be a cow or
a bull. The goat sacrifice had served to dissolve the bonds between the
initiate and the senior healer, the cow or bull sacrifice symbolizes the final

stage of the initiate's journey and culminates in her evolution as a full-fledged healer by forging the bond between the initiate and the ancestors.

In the dream, the cow is accompanied by three unknown visitors. For Ntombi, these suggest a visitation from her ancestors. Marie-Louise von Franz (1970) commented on unknown visitors in dreams and fairy tales as often being representative of divine beings or of God and bringers of gifts. Ntombi is responsive to the visitors and the gift of the cow, which hints at the possible integration of these aspects.

This dream the image of the cow is remarkably transformed compared to the distorted cow image in the first dream (chapter 5). The deeper amplification of the symbol of the cow reveals it to be archetypally the symbol of the great mother, an aspect of the foundation of life as well as representative of the goddesses through the ages. The amplification of the cow symbolism with respect to ancient Egyptian mythology is applicable given the appearance of the cow in the dream with the golden disk. In the Egyptian pantheon, Isis and Hathor are represented as a cow. Depictions of Hathor with the solar disc between her horns reflect the image of the cow in the dream. Hera, wife of Zeus, saved her life by changing into a cow, and in India cows are venerated and held sacred. The domesticated cow is the producer of milk and nourishment.

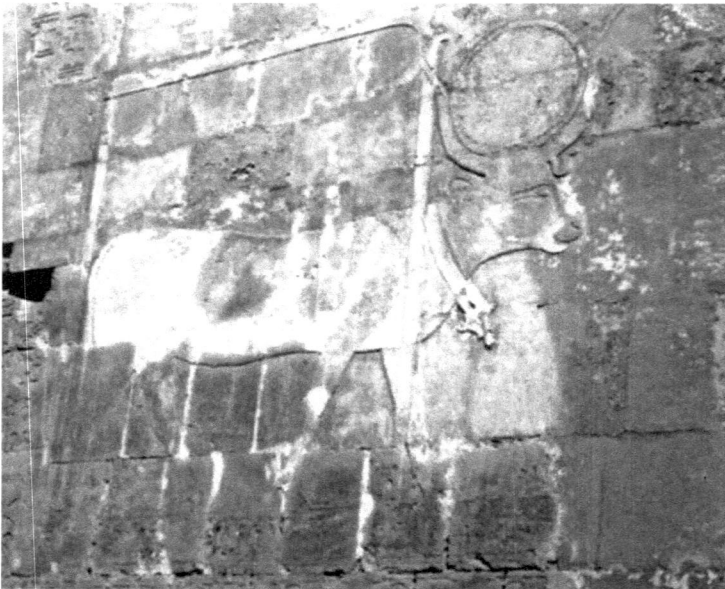

Figure 32. Hathor with sun disk, Temple of Hathor, Luxor, Egypt

The cow, as an image of the mother goddess, the cosmic maternal principle, and the feminine principle of fertility, carries on her head a golden disk. The disk is a symbol of the Self par excellence, and the gold signifies that which is of the highest value. Here, this particular symbol of the Self seems to reflect that aspect of the totality, as a sun disk is a symbol of consciousness and a new dawn. The symbol of the sun or the golden disk is immense. As Jung (1944) elaborated: "The sun is the "symbol of the unity of the self" and "an image of God" (para. 108, 445). In the Egyptian pantheon, the sun is the element of the sun god, Ra, and of Horus as the "rising sun, the enlightener" (see Jung 1954b, para. 361, fn. 13; for further discussion of the symbol of the sun disk, the Mithraic liturgy, and the sun wheel, see Jung 1952b).

In the dream, the golden disk or sun is carried in the horns of the cow, the feminine aspect and the maternal foundation of life. The horns further suggest something that is emerging, pointing upward, and their crescent shape evokes the lunar principle. This dream image suggests a *coniunctio,* a coming together of the upper and the lower realms, the cow and the sun disk, Sol and Lunar, masculine and feminine.

In the African worldview the cow carries sacred numinosity and is referred to as "god with the wet nose." The cow symbolizes the connection or bridge to the sacred. Cows are said to occupy the space between the living and the living dead, the ancestors. It is at the moment of the sacrifice of the cow that the ancestors are said to express their willingness to accept the new healer or to show their displeasure and refusal. The dream seems to suggest to the dreamer the task that Jung (1961a) described as that of converting instinctual impulses into religious activity.

The black and white coloring of the cow in Ntombi's dream embodies opposites. The quaternity of the two men and two women (including the dreamer) suggest a totality, a wholeness that in the symbolism of the four enters into consciousness as the dreamer "awakes" in the dream.

At times, the dream of the initiate may indicate that the final sacrificial animal is a bull as a dream of an initiate illustrates:

> *A small herd of sacred bulls are secured in a kraal. As I approach,*
> *one breaks free from the herd and runs through the gate. He is*
> *vibrant and full of energy. A deep brown color with a white streak*
> *in his face. I know that is how my bull will look.*

On the individual level, the difference between the cow or bull seems to compensate for a too strong masculine or feminine energy in the initiate. The bull is a symbol of masculine generative power, creative fecundity, potency, strength, and fertility. Bull symbolism appears in the Egyptian pantheon in the forms of the bull gods, including Apis, Buchis (the holy white bull), and Min. The bull is venerated in India as the bull Indras in the Rigveda, particularly for the strength and the piercing quality of their horns.

The symbolic range of the bull, like the cow, is immense and embodies solar and lunar elements as well as all four elements of nature: its deep bellow symbolizing thunder, its huge body the solidity of earth, its virility associated with sun, and crescent horns with the moon (de Vries, 1974). The flooding of the Nile in Egypt and the Tigris in Mesopotamia are the result of the union between the bull god and cow goddess of Mother Earth. Shiva temples have Nandi and his adoring bull facing the inner sanctum, known as the great inseminator. Mothers-to-be would touch his testicles to get pregnant. Sacrifice of the bull crosses many mythologies, including that of ancient Greece, where on the island of Kos, the bull is said to choose himself for the sacrifice by bowing his head. The sacrifice contains in it the accessing of the mana of the animal, a spiritualization of instinct. Curative and

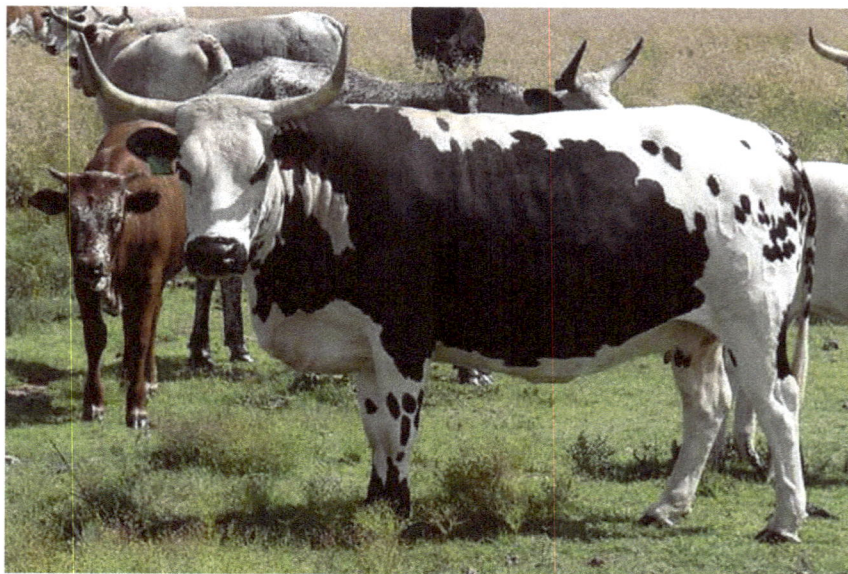

Figure 33. The *Nguni* cow is indigenous to South Africa and resembles the cow in the dream as well as the image of Hathor (Figure 32)

restorative plants are said grow from the blood of the sacrificed bull in the Mithraic myth (Hannah, 2006).

The Cow or Bull Sacrifice

This final sacrifice is the most auspicious and celebrated of all the rituals. It is this ceremony that marks the emergence of the new healer. Healers will travel far distances and at great personal expense in order to attend this final sacrifice. This is the graduation ceremony, which functions to solidify the bond between the initiate and the ancestors. It is called *ukuphothula,* the final "taking-home" ceremony.

The first part is the separation of the ancestors. The healers explain that during the initial stages of the initiation, the healer and initiate work closely together and their respective ancestors are like one. This ceremony functions to separate the healer's ancestors from the initiate's ancestors. As Ntombi reflected, "our ancestors were united, now we must divide them to see if I can stand on my own." This is not unlike the analytical process where the patient becomes more autonomous or, in the case of an analysand, begins to treat patients.

The second part of the ceremony is the induction ceremony. This process is conducted with extreme seriousness and reverence, as the initiate is now introduced to the ancestors and is welcomed into the ranks of the healers in the new identity as healer. The unfolding of this ritual has extreme emotional, psychological, spiritual, and physical implications for the *thwasa.* After dreaming her cow or bull, she is then expected to find the animal in actuality and to develop a relationship with the animal. The characteristic of the animal's nature often reflects the instinctual nature of the initiate. An initiate explained:

> I have to wait until the dream comes. The dream will tell me if I need to find a cow or a bull. In the dream I will be shown exactly the animal that I need to find. Like in my dream, I saw the bull. I saw his colors, deep brown with a white mark between his eyes. When I wake, I have to now go and find this bull. It took many weeks until I found exactly the bull from my dreams. When I found him, it was like he recognized me, too.

The animal becomes, in a way, the embodiment of the ancestral spirit of the initiate. The sacrifice requires an exchange, in that something of the animal is given to the initiate and, in turn, an aspect of the initiate is sacrificed. As a healer explained:

> At that time, that moment before the sacrifice, I will communicate with the bull and ask permission for the sacrifice. At that moment, I can no longer tell the difference between me and the animal. I am the animal and the animal is me. I am not only sacrificing the bull but also myself.

Von Franz (1998) explained the psychological value of the sacrifice as the principle of individuation wherein the ego submits to a higher inner authority:

> The central significance of the sacrifice . . . is *the* possibility for the ego to experience a superior presence, the reality of the Self . . . For the Self it is a moment in time when it can enter into us, and so pass from a condition of unconsciousness into consciousness, from potentiality into actuality. It is . . . the moment when the "unknown god" in us becomes conscious, thereby becoming at the same time human. (p. 229)

For the African healer, the honoring of the sacrifice manifests in the healing energy. These sacrifices cannot be separated from the healing. They are sacred rites, *opera divinum*, with the purpose of placing the individual in direct contact with ancestral energies. Psychologically, we could say that this places the individual in direct contact with the autonomous reality of the objective psyche.

The Cow or Bull and the Number Four

The significance of the number symbolism embedded in the stages of the initiation rituals is not immediately apparent to the casual observer. However, after one has participated in and officiated over many of these initiations, the timing and the number of days becomes clear.

The four is central to the final sacrifice of the bull or the cow. For the *thwasa,* the cow or the bull ceremony often takes place over four days with no sleep or rest. Four, or the four aspect of one, is a manifestation of symmetry, a quaternity. Four suggests completion (von Franz, 1974): the four phases of the moon, four weeks in a month, four seasons of the year, and four directions of the compass; the four basic elements—earth, water, fire, ether; and the four functions of consciousness—thinking, feeling, intuition, and sensation.

With the number four we reach a definite limit beyond which something new begins. Four is the archetypal background by which ego consciousness is structured (Apt, 2005). After this four-day ceremony, the new healer is introduced to the community and is able to function autonomously and begin training initiates.

Similarly the four holds a position of outstanding symbolic meaning within Jungian psychology. Von Franz (1974) reflected on "the vast psychological significance of the number four," and she stated unequivocally:

> The fact that mankind's repeated attempts to establish an orientation toward wholeness possess a quaternity structure appears to correspond to an archetypal psychic structural predisposition in man. . . . In all models of the universe and concepts of the divine . . . a fourfold structure dominates. . . . The number four remained . . . *the* number of the elements, aggregate states, alchemical steps, temperaments and so forth. . . . (p. 115)

This experience reflects von Franz's comment: "the numerical rhythms one, two, three, and four . . . *acquire an especially decisive significance when they appear as the structural characteristics of the Self symbol,* in the form of cosmic models and divine symbols" (1974, p. 124). In other words, each number—one, two, three, four—represents a totality in itself; that is, each number symbolizes a different aspect of the archetype of the Self.

We can recall that for the initiate, each number, in combination with each sacrifice, embodies a numinous development that ultimately leads to the transformation of initiate into healer. In a psychological sense, each stage of the initiation in relation to the number symbolism suggests different levels of development in consciousness.

Von Franz (1974) explains that the development in consciousness from the three to the four requires a shift from "a purely imaginary standpoint" to one in which there is an actual experience and participation. In other words, at this juncture there is a materialization of spirit as well as a spiritualization of matter. To quote von Franz (1974):

> In a curiously retrograde manner the number four brings us, once again, back to the *unus mundus*. As a consequence of the step to four, our mental processes no longer revolve about intellectual theorizations, but partake of the creative adventure of "realizations in the act of becoming." (p. 131)

The healers emphasize the necessity of the time frame of each of the ceremonies contributes to the transformation of the initiate. They maintain, and it has been my experience, that it is only through the prolonged process of the ceremonies that a transformation of consciousness is possible. As von Franz (1974) noted that "it is therefore not surprising that the step from three to four involves particular difficulties for it is bound up with painful insights" (p. 129). This is true of the final four-day ceremony, as Jung (1958b) elaborates:

> By unfolding into the four it acquires distinct characteristics and can therefore be known. . . . So long as a thing is in the unconscious it has no recognizable qualities . . . But as soon as the unconscious content enters the sphere of consciousness it has already split into the "four." (para. 774)

As this final ceremony heralds the emergence of the fully fledged healer, the alchemical concept of the *quinta essenia* in relation to the four is relevant. Von Franz (1974) explains that the fifth

> is not additively joined onto the first four as a fifth element, but represents the most refined, spiritually imaginable unity of the four elements. It is either initially present in and extracted from them or produced by the circulation of these elements among one another (p. 121).

This seems to reflect the development of healing abilities in the healer after the four-day ceremony. To wit, the healing energy symbolizes, so to say, the culmination of the initiation process—the refined essence. This quintessence is represented by the quincunx, the center of the four (⁙). The quincunx thus holds the central position as a mediator between the pair of opposites that comprise the four. In this aspect, the five as the quintessence suggests that which is extracted from the four, or the spiritual unity of the four, here represented by the fully fledged healer.

This final sacrifice is pregnant with expectation. It marks the transition toward transformation and, if successful, the birth of a new healer. After this sacrifice, the *thwasa* is separated and secluded from the community. This is a time of contemplation as Ntombi reflected:

> During the seclusion I became aware of the channel to the ancestors. Somehow I had a sense that they were pleased with my development. I was also aware of a sense of anticipation and responsibility. I knew that when I emerged from the seclusion, I would now carry the mantle of the healer.

Ntombi's evolution was dependent on her supreme concentration and fidelity to the rituals as a whole and to this final sacrifice in particular. The death of the animal and the honoring of the animal in death attest to the bond that develops between the initiate and the animal. By observing the ritual, following it, and listening to its truth, Ntombi learned the will of the gods, or psychologically, the Self. In so doing, both undergo a transformation in that there is a reciprocal exchange between consciousness and the unconscious.

Chapter 9
Umbilini:
Union of Opposites

My spirit has been healed.
—Ntombi

A feature of the alchemical work is the creation of a hermetically sealed vessel, symbolic of a psychic attitude that is capable of holding the tension of opposing elements or opposites until something transforms. For the healer, this is the *umbilini,* the core, like an umbilicus where body and soul unite. The *umbilini* is "awakened" in the vessel of the initiation, and it is this phenomenon that connects the healer to the ancestors. What is required psychologically is a strong ego consciousness that is open to what Marie-Louise von Franz (1997a) called "a visit from the gods" (p. 73). This "visit from the gods" is poignantly illustrated by a unique aspect to the calling referred to in chapter 3.

Going under the Water

The complexity of the process with Ntombi was highlighted with an added dimension to her initiatory experience that neither Ntombi nor I had anticipated, which further exemplifies the ego's awakening to the Self. Not all the initiates are required to undergo this aspect of the initiation. It seems that the differences lie in the individual destinies of the initiates. According to the Zulu healers:

The *sangoma* draws knowledge from the hidden lake. There is a huge unseen lake somewhere in the spirit world where all the knowledge of the universe, past, present, and future, is to be found: A treasure house of knowledge. The carrier of this knowledge is *Inkanyambo*, the ancestral snake of the Zulu people. (Mutwa, 1996, p. 124)

Ntombi's dreams and visions during her seclusion mentioned above seemed to demand that she undergo the underwater initiation. She commented: "The river ceremony was the most difficult for me. I was always scared of the water. We are told many do not return from under the water." Ntombi shared the following account:

I was very ill. My body hurt all over. I had been to doctors; no one could help. I was feverish, lying at the doorway, too weak to move. Then I heard a rustling to my left. A little white bird was coming towards me. She came right up to me and whispered in my ear. I felt her breath in my ear, and I could get up. I had the strength to walk, to follow her. I followed her to the great river. My feet followed her, and we went under to the bottom. I looked there, and I saw a huge dragon-like snake. She was white with many breasts coming towards me. There were many snakes under the water and a light so I could see clearly. The snakes were all suckled by the huge one.

She was quite terrifying, with horns on her head and a light that seemed to shine from inside her head. Her eyes burnt with fire. I felt my body coming apart, coming apart in pieces and dissolving. When I came together again, my body came together again, all the snakes were now one, and she was now many colors and shining. In the stones she showed me all the medicines. I do not know how long I was there, but when I returned, the people thought I had died or drowned. But I returned and I had the medicines and the knowledge, the secret knowledge.

At the time that Ntombi related this account to me, I had the following dream:

I am in my healing room, meditating. Through the upper left-hand window, a huge snake enters. It is a male with a huge horned head. Its body is covered in scales that are arranged in clearly defined geometric patterns that remind me of mandalas. It enters the room and slithers down the wall, coiling around me as I sit on the floor. I feel a mixture of fear and awe. It births a young snake from each of the geometric designs—live births, not from eggs. The young all merge into one huge snake, a female snake.

Jung (1961a) gave a description of one of his own experiences of the serpent in an active imagination, one that bears a remarkable similarity to Ntombi's account. During the period when Jung separated from Freud, Jung seemed to undergo his own *nigredo*, which led to his confrontation with the unconscious and his first encounter with Elijah and Salome.[17] Through this direct encounter with the unconscious, Jung gained an awareness of the reality and autonomy of the objective psyche. During his "meeting" with Elijah and Salome, Jung wrote: "They had a black serpent living with them which displayed an unmistakable fondness for me" (1961a, p. 206). Jung explained that "the serpent is the personification of the tendency to go into the depths and to deliver oneself over to the alluring world of shadows (1989, p. 103). Jung continued in relation to the serpent, "I saw the snake approach me. She came close and began to encircle me and press me in her coils … in agony and the struggle, I sweated so profusely that the water flowed down on all sides of me" (1989, p. 104).

"Going under the water" can be understood psychologically as a deep introversion, an immersion into the unfathomable depths of the collective unconscious, where dream and fantasy states, as well as active imagination, are the "dissolving waters." Ntombi described the experience as one of drowning under the water; von Franz (1997c) noted that "everyone who starts an analysis drowns within her own imaginative activity" (p. 53). In alchemy this stage of drowning or *dissolutio* (dissolution) is a necessary precursor to transformation, which is not possible until the original *prima materia* has dissolved. Von Franz (1980a) explained that often the alchemical work begins with liquefaction (see chapter 6). In this alchemical operation, the fixed or rigidified solid of the *prima materia* is turned into liquid in order to undo the *prima materia* which often has hardened or solidified in a wrong way . . . this is the equivalent of a dissolution of the personality . . . through which the creative content of the unconscious can emerge . . . the liquefying process is necessary in order to approach the layer where the unconscious can come up and speak. (p. 196)

Active Imagination and *Mundus imaginalis*

The quality of the "under the water" experience evokes the quality of the active imagination described by Jung, von Franz, Hannah, and others. Jung (1955–56) explained the different stages of the active imagination process, which can take place spontaneously or be actively induced (para. 706). Jung stressed that at a certain point in an active imagination it is necessary to move from a passive observation of images to a conscious participation in the events unfolding in order to integrate the contents of the unconscious. As Barbara Hannah (1981) informs us: "The greatest use of active imagination is to put us . . . into harmony with the Tao so that the right things may happen around us" (p. 14).

It is under the water that Ntombi encounters and engages with the primordial aspect of the autonomous psyche in the form of the snake. It is here that she is confronted with an aspect of the Self and awakens to her healing abilities.

In Ntombi's description, she starts out in a passive state and is approached by the white bird, an experience that seems to resemble the waking dream or vision state. As such, her account hints at the idea of the *mundus imaginalis*, a term coined by Henry Corbin (1964). This concept was intended to encapsulate the idea of that intermediary state between waking and sleeping, or "a place out of place." These experiences of going under the water present the Western mind with the challenge of unifying thinking and being, which would take us beyond the physical world. As Corbin (1964) described:

We realize immediately that we are no longer confined to the dilemma of thought and extension, to the schema of a cosmology and a gnoseology restricted to the empirical world and the world of abstract intellect. Between them there is a world that is both intermediary and intermediate . . . the world of image, the *mundus imaginalis*; a world that is ontologically as real as the world of the senses and that of the intellect . . . represented by a world possessing extension and dimension, figures and colors . . . that are the objects of the psycho-spiritual senses. (p. 5)

For the healer there is an added dimension. The underwater phenomenon is a direct inner experience of the "ancestor of the water" (chapter 3), an archetypal ontological being in possession of healing knowledge. This form of initiation is seen as the most auspicious as well as the most dangerous, in that many are said never to return, which can imply an actual death or falling into an inflation and identification with the unconscious psyche.

Amplification of Symbols

There are a number of symbols that could be amplified this account. I will limit myself to the main images and a selection of amplifications that have direct implications for the initiation process: the water, the messenger (in the form of a bird), and particularly, the snake.

The Water

Water is the *prima materia* from which all life began, and psychologically, it symbolizes the creative fecundity of the unconscious psyche. The rivers, the veins of Mother Earth, and images of divine waters flow through most mythologies that describe accounts of how the great waters came to earth, such as the four rivers of paradise and the seven rivers in Vedic mythology. In ancient Greek, Chinese, and Indian myths the dead are believed to continue to live in the groundwater under the earth, in large underground rivers such as the Acheron, the river of woe, and the Cocytus, the river of wailing.

Encounters with otherworldly beings during a night sea journey are often central motifs in resurrection and individuation myths. In ancient

Egyptian mythology, the souls of the dead sail through the Amduat, the underworld, where they encounter a number of challenges, the most perilous being the serpent Apophis, and Jonah encounters the whale on his journey toward transformation. The Hindus scatter the ashes of the dead on the waters, symbolizing a redeeming dissolution and a return to the primal ocean.

Water is associated with the nocturnal states of the soul, the womb, creativity, fertility, regeneration, and the source of life. As a threshold between worlds, between the living and the dead, consciousness and the unconscious, water is where the physical and spiritual worlds merge. Water is the place of suspension where the concrete can become fluid and the spirit manifest.

In alchemy and in the writings of Zosimos, we find the description of the divine waters, *hydro theios*, "the wonder-working water, which is both water and spirit, and kills and vivifies" (Jung, 1954e, para.135). The amplification of the divine waters reflects the primeval waters and the source of life, which is immanent in everything and which contains opposites: masculine and feminine, life and death. Neumann (1954) spoke of the state of being under the water as dissolution or a "sinking back into the pleroma, a self-surrender" (p. 37). He noted that this is not so much a regression, but a return to the creative matrix with the dissolution of the ego.

As is evident from the above account of Ntombi, "going under the water" entails a death and rebirth journey. By entering into the depths of the unconscious, she undergoes a rebirthing experience and reemerges transformed. Von Franz (1984) elaborated that the symbolism of water in dreams can have a negative meaning, such as being inundated by flood, or it can have a vivifying effect, bringing a new understanding to a stagnant problem in the outer life, after which the channel to the unconscious flows once again.

The Messenger

Ntombi is led to the water by the white bird. The bird is a symbol pregnant with meaning and can be amplified as the messenger of the unconscious and of the gods. To the ancient Greeks the actions of birds were seen as prophecies (from the Greek etymology for Ornithomancy), and the ancient

Romans observed the flight of the birds in order to foretell the will of the gods. The bird is the link between heaven and earth and symbolizes the soul, for example, the Egyptian Ba-soul, the mercurial winged god of alchemy, and the white dove of the Holy Spirit. Ancient shamans flew on birds or transformed into winged creatures. The archetype of the bird is most often connected to the spiritual world, an image of the divine or the beyond. Psychologically, the bird suggests notions or inspirations that "fly" up from the unconscious, including flights of ideas, which can also suggest unwanted distractions. In the natural world bird song wakes us in the morning and calls us back to consciousness.

Within the African tradition, the bird is a manifestation of the ancestors. At the very least, this symbol carries a message from the unconscious that seeks to break through or ascend into consciousness. Jung (1961a) described his vision of the white bird in 1912 that appeared while he sat at the table with his children; he recognized the *"visitation* as an unusual activation of the unconscious" (p. 195).

The white color of the bird is significant. White is associated with magical and spiritual ideas as well as death, a departure from something, annihilation, and detachment. The color white can suggest that which cannot be touched, such as a white heat. Psychologically, this could indicate a dangerous autonomous unconscious eruption. White is also associated with new life, a transition to something new, purity and immortality. White symbolizes a life giving aspect of the unconscious, a window to eternity, a space for that which is not yet to emerge (Apt, 2005). Both aspects of the amplification of the color white—to life and to death—are applicable here (see also chapter 6). The attitude of Ntombi to the bird in her account reflects Jung's recommendation that if something appears during active imagination, follow it (in Hannah, 1981). In following the bird, in honoring the manifestation of the unconscious, Ntombi meets *Inkanyambo*, the ancestral snake.

The Horned Snake

Within the African cosmology, the snake is one of the most feared and powerful forms of the ancestors. Psychologically, the snake is one of the most pregnant symbols of the unconscious, at times seen as standing for the unconscious itself, and thus archetypal in nature. Amplifications of the snake symbolism can continue eternally. I will endeavor to do justice to this symbol, as it is one of my personal and most potent ancestral forms. I have had a number of encounters with snakes, mostly in a helpful way.

One incident came to mind as I was compiling this section. I was preparing to leave for my practice one morning. As is often the case, I was rushing, not wanting to be late for my first appointment. I opened my door and sitting on the threshold on the other side of the screen door was a fully grown golden cobra. At the sound of the door opening, she raised her head with hood flared and looked straight at me. I knew that there was no way I would be able to get around her; she was not going anywhere.

I sat on the floor, a little distance away, and we watched each other. I had to let go of my schedule and time frame and just sit until she decided what to do. She made no move to enter the house or to leave. After a full fifteen minutes, she dipped her head as if in salutation and slowly slithered off into the bush. I could now leave. A few minutes later, on the road not far from my home, I passed a fatal accident where a truck had overturned and five cars had been involved. The ambulances and police had just arrived on the scene. Of course, I gave silent thanks to this ancestral spirit as perhaps, had I left in my usual hurry and driving too fast, I just may have been involved in the accident.

Psychologically, the presence of the snake in dreams, visions, and active imaginations can be symbolic of an aspect of the Self. As Jung (1951) elucidated, the snake corresponds to "the collective unconscious and . . . instinct, seems to possess a peculiar wisdom of its own and a knowledge that is often felt to be supernatural" (para. 370). In this sense, the snake also stands for the Self.

The snake is frequently the guardian of treasure, with the capacity for eternal renewal, the agency of activation, and regeneration, often symbolized by the ancient image of the *uroboros*. In African mythology the presence of the snake indicates a visitation from the ancestors and the awareness that a process of transformation is occurring. Initially, as in dreams and in the above account, the snake appears as an ambivalent figure. This suggests that first a terrifying manifestation must take place in order to obtain that which is of value. Once an awareness of the meaning of the visitation has been understood, the snake becomes an ally.

Von Franz (1980a) noted that one often meets the antagonistic aspect of the collective unconscious in this symbol, such as the dark transpersonal power of Set and the Apophis serpent (p. 51). She warns that the weak or immature or inflated ego can be destroyed by this archetypal energy. Neumann (1954) explains that it is necessary for the ego's position to be strengthened through the rituals, symbolic dismemberments, and reintegration, as only then can such energy can be assimilated and appropriated in consciousness, eventually becoming a function of the ego. This reflects Ntombi's process in that this new aspect of her initiation emerged after she had completed the previous stages during which her ego consciousness had been both strengthened and humbled enough in order to encounter the numinous unconscious under the water and to return with the healing knowledge.

The snake is the mediator of hidden processes of transformation and rebirth, symbolically seen as having power over life and death and the shedding of its skin is symbolic of immortality, fertility, and potency (de Vries, 1974). Snakes often arouse fear as they are said to embody the spirits of the dead. Psychologically, this is symbolic of the enigmatic and frightening aspect of the unconscious psyche. The snake often enters a dream or vision when the Self urgently needs to be heard. This underlies the "under the water" initiation, where the encounter with the snake symbolizes the archetype of the ancestor of the water. Barbara Hannah (2006), in her lectures on the archetypal symbolism of animals, noted in relation to the snake:

> It is absolutely necessary to do the things that interest the gods, one of the hardest things in the process of individuation, and it is just here that the snake is our best hope, for it represents that instinct which knows what interests the gods and makes us do it . . . if we can listen to the snake and hear its voice, it will whisper this secret to us, and that is why it is so universally recognized as a divinity, or . . . as a mediator between the divine and man . . . it is only from great effort of consciousness that the serpent solution will be constellated. (p. 236)

Jung (1952b) commented on the snake as the relentless death-dealing aspect of nature, the instinctual psyche with its "sudden and unexpected manifestations, its painful and dangerous [and helpful] interventions in our affairs and its frightening affects" (para. 580). The snake is the theriomorphic form of many deities, including Zeus, Apollo, Persephone, Hades, Isis, Kali,

Shakti, and the Kundalini. It embodies the opposites, dark and cold, but also warmth and radiance, danger and healing; it is able to accomplish miracle cures and appears in most indigenous mythologies from the Aborigines of Australia to those of India, Africa, and North and South America.

Von Franz (in Jung, 2008) gave a detailed account of the symbolism of the snake. With deep understanding von Franz explained that the snake belongs to the chthonic female elements in opposition to the spiritual male world. It embodies a dual symbolism as primal enemy of the upper-world gods: Gaia as earth goddess creates the half-snake titans who wrestle with Zeus, the leviathan that is the antagonist of Jehovah. The snake resembles the basilisk, a legendary reptile thought to be the king of serpents, whose defeat heralds the beginning of many heroic legends. The snake is the vital, instinctual drive, the unconscious dark side, with its antinomy of healing. Its appearance in dreams can often signal healing and return of vital power. The snake is also the instinct that is the catalyst toward a development in consciousness and toward individuation, for example, the snake in Eden who entices Eve to take a step toward consciousness.

The souls of the dead live on in the chthonic snake gods as inhabitants of the underworld, where they become the guardians of the treasure, possessor of the herbs of life with which they can reawaken the dead. The snake further embodies the concept of time as the image of the uroboros and is associated with Aion, the god of eternal duration. The many-breasted snake in Ntombi's account evokes an association to the image of Diana of Ephesus as the life-giving fertility symbol, and also to the creative capacity of the objective psyche. Thus, through this glimpse into the rich symbolism of the snake, we can begin to grasp the reverence for the snake, which brought about its apotheosis in the African healing cosmogony and where the snake emerges most impressively in this aspect of the initiation.

Ntombi described a light and the glowing eyes of the snake that burn despite being under the water. This suggests the *lapis philosophorum* or the diamond of higher consciousness, the inner light, and the secret fire that dwells in the depths of the earth. The snake and its relation to the *lapis*, the stone, is central in the alchemical opus, wherein the poison of the snake turns into the ultimate medicine. Jung (1944) described the snake symbol as that which encompasses, guards, and gestates the treasures of the Self, the symbol of secret wisdom, the one who reveals the hidden knowledge (para. 356). As in the Gnostic tenets, snake wisdom is the knowledge coming

148

from nature itself, from inner experience. This is further symbolized by the white snake in Ntombi's vision as the spiritual serpent, bringing secret knowledge, wisdom, and revelation.

Von Franz (1997c) commented on the snake imagery in relation to inner life. She noted that if one stays with the introversion long enough, something changes, the flood of the unconscious recedes and something is born within, such as a realization of the Self. The individual returns with healing capacity. Meier (1989) noted that in the Gilgamesh epic, the snake was said to dwell in the water and to eat the herb of life. This seems reflective of the "under the water" account in that Ntombi, having gone through a meditative work with the snake in the unconscious as well as a death and inner resurrection experience, returns with the healing knowledge.

A pertinent amplification of the snake symbolism for the theme of this work is the association with the Greek god Asclepius, or Hermes or Mercurius and the symbol of the caduceus—the rod entwined by two serpents. The image often symbolizes the *coniunctio* of consciousness and the unconscious. In ancient Greek mythology, Asclepius was worshipped near the healing waters. He learned the art of healing from the centaur

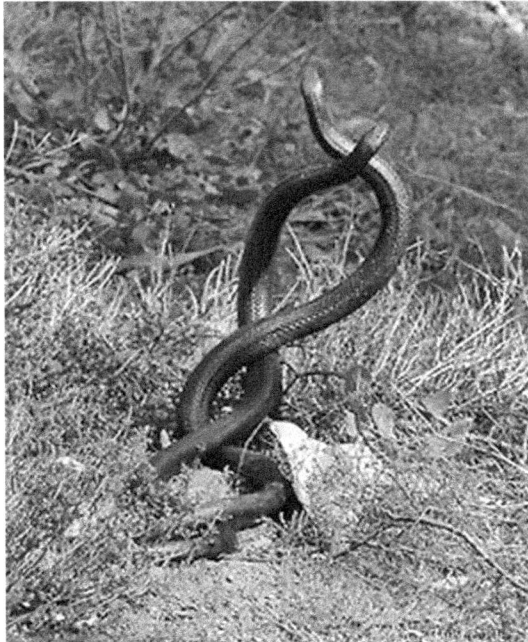

Figure 34: Attending an initiation I came across these two entwined snakes on the pathway

Chiron, who had been wounded by Heracles and is thus an image of the wounded healer archetype. Asclepius was said to embody opposites with both mantic and chthonic properties. As a male god, he was also a god of fertility in that he was said to have borne many children (Meier, 1989). This reflects again the experiences of Ntombi under the water and the descriptions of the many snakes born of the one snake. Thus the theme of the healing arts associated with the snake and the water is woven throughout our ancient knowledge.

In Ntombi's vision and my dream, the snake is horned and resembles the dragon of the alchemists. Jung (1944) described the alchemist's vision of dragons and creatures within the retort as images of the inner workings of the unconscious psyche. The dragon embodies a chthonic energy, which suggests an archetypal phenomenon of unrealized proportions, or psychologically, the experience of being gripped by something autonomous, potentially overpowering, and yet fascinating. Von Franz (1980a) observed that "snakes and dragons are common representations, in mythology and dreams, of the impersonal spirit of the unconscious" (p. 243).

Jung provided a detailed account of the connection between the dragon motif, the idea of transformation, and the symbolism of the alchemical Mercurius. Mercurius was for the alchemist the symbol of the "mysterious transforming substance" that embodied opposites. As Jung (1944) outlined:

> It is of the essence of the transforming substance to be on the one hand extremely common, even contemptible (this expressed in the qualities it shares with the devil, such as serpent, dragon . . .), but on the other hand to mean something of great value, not to say divine. (para. 173)

Under the water, Ntombi meets a frightening chthonic being that is initially threatening and later undergoes a transformation, revealing its antinomy, in that it is the keeper of the healing knowledge. This is further symbolized by the image of the many snakes coming together in a unified being, which suggests a transformation taking place. The "under the water" phenomenon is that which dissolves the boundary between consciousness and the unconscious, between spirit and matter. It is this realm that Ntombi is able to receive healing knowledge and to embrace her calling. As Jung (1944) noted with respect to the alchemical rites:

The symbolism of the rites of renewal, if taken seriously, points far beyond the merely archaic and infantile to man's innate psychic disposition, which is the result and deposit of all ancestral life right down to the animal level—hence the ancestor and animal symbolism. The rites are attempts to abolish the separation between the conscious mind and the unconscious, the real source of life, and to bring about a reunion of the individual with the native soil of his inherited, instinctive makeup. (para. 174)

This initiatory experience, psychologically, can be conceptualized as a healing through the contact with an aspect of the Self, an aspect of the process of individuation. This is the process that forces one to step out of daily life into contemplation, and doing so stimulates the flow of the unconscious waters, or symbolically, going under the water.

Ntombi further described an experience of dismemberment under the water, a process of fragmentation and dissolution, which leads to differentiation and renewal (see also chapter 6). Many creation myths

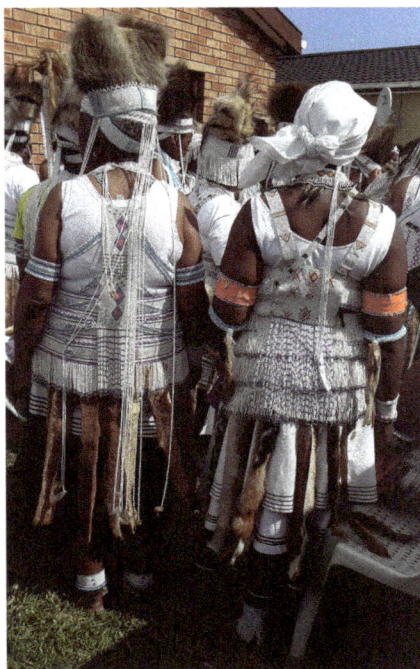

Figure 35. The healers gather to await the return of the initiate at the water ceremony

describe the archetypal process of the dismemberment of the primordial being preceding transformation. This theme is found in the myths of ancient Greece, Babylonia, India, and Egypt, and in Jewish mysticism and the Christian Eucharist. Dismemberment is characteristic of most shamanic traditions from Asia to Siberia, Australia and Africa, and in the Indo-Tibetan and Native American cultures. Psychologically, dismemberment is the death of an aspect of the ego, or a setting aside of ego-driven desires, before a transformation and rebirth.

Hero Archetype and the Archetype of Initiation

This form of the initiation can be amplified as an expression of the hero archetype and archetype of initiation (Campbell, 1968). It is an image of the hero's journey in that it is undertaken alone, it is considered dangerous; many do not return, but those that do are considered to be the most auspicious of the healers. Campbell (1968) wrote:

> The hero ventures forth from the world of common day into a region of supernatural wonder. Fabulous forces are there encountered and a decisive victory is won: the hero comes back from this mysterious adventure with the power to bestow a boon on his fellow man. (p. 30)

The above description describes Ntombi's experience in the the "under water" initiation. Initially, Ntombi describes a period of illness and isolation. This is followed by the calling to go "under the water," to cross a threshold between the known and the unknown. The entry into the water is akin to a death/rebirth image. The initiate is swallowed into an unknown world and is thought to have died. The passage across this threshold is a form of self-annihilation and a turning inward before the rebirth. Under the water, Ntombi faced a number of trials and confrontations, the biggest of which is the confrontation with the snake under whose belly lies the healing medicines. In facing the snake, an enantiodromia occurs where the potentially destructive power of the snake transforms, the snake becomes an ally of the initiate and permits the acquisition of healing medicines. At this time, the initiate is exposed to the greatest risk. That many do not return reflects the danger of the confrontation with the archetypes of the objective psyche. Jung (1952b) explained that the god

> first appears in hostile form . . . with whom the hero has to wrestle . . . The onslaught of the instinct then becomes an experience of divinity, provided that man does not succumb to it and follow it blindly, but defends his humanity against the animal nature of the divine power. (para. 524)

In many accounts, healers also describe a transformation that takes place in the snake once the healing gifts have been obtained. The snakes then become very beautiful, accompanied by a feeling in the initiate of wanting to stay under the water. Often the initiates are told not to look back at the snake once they have claimed the medicine. Here the initiate is warned against the hypnotic powers of the unconscious forces and a regressive attachment to the underworld, with a submersion in the unconscious.

The hero archetype is representative of the pattern of detachment from the collective and thus the individuation process. The individuation process, as noted by Jung (1923) essentially births the "development of the psychological individual as a differentiated being from the general collective psychology" (para. 757). The entry into the water and the return symbolizes the descent into the unconscious and the emergence from it. For Jung (1944)

> the purpose of the descent as universally exemplified in the myth of the hero is to show that only in the region of danger (the watery abyss, cavern, forest . . .) can one find the "treasure hard to obtain" . . . (the jewel, virgin, life potion, victory over death) (para. 438)

Jung (1966) continued, pointing to the danger of venturing into the unconscious and thereby acquiring new consciousness:

> It is precisely the strongest and the best man among the people, the hero, who gives way to the regressive longing and deliberately exposes himself to the danger of being devoured by the monster of the maternal abyss. He is, however, a hero only because in the final reckoning he does not allow himself to be devoured. (para. 477)

The rituals and ceremonies provide a powerful temenos for the constellation of numinous psychic energies that is often lacking in a more one-sided rational worldview. Campbell (1968) noted that clusters of symbols operate in rituals and have the power to carry the spirit forward to new experiences; they seem to bridge the divide between conscious states and unconscious material. This has the effect of enlarging and unifying the personality. In the *thwasa*, this development is seen internally in the communication with the ancestors and externally in terms of a greater capacity for healing. Thus the symbol of the hero myth, as Neumann (1954) explained, is a symbol of an ego able to relate to the unconscious content actively and willingly. The hero archetype therefore is the archetype that underscores the rites of passage that populate indigenous cultures and some religious systems still today.

An important differentiation needs to be highlighted with respect to the hero archetype and archetype of initiation. Henderson and Oakes (1963) clarified that the heroic mode of behavior, having accomplished its purpose of helping the ego overcome the inertia of the unconscious, must be replaced with another myth, whereby consciousness of the ego is transformed into consciousness of the Self. In my experience, the African healing initiation focused on in this work is a living modern image of the archetype of initiation.

Initially, the journey under the water requires the heroic effort of the ego to overcome fear and to embark on the initiation journey. Then one is called to turn inward and to withdraw, as the word *initiation* ("to enter into") implies. Heroic actions are no longer required but rather what is required is submission. This often involves a descent into the underworld, the unconscious, the creative matrix of the *prima materia*, the fertility of nature.

The feat achieved by Ntombi in going under the water is in being able to encounter the annihilating potential of the uroboric snake without being devoured. In the process of the calling, this begins with being overwhelmed by the energies of the objective psyche and develops toward an ability to relate to and negotiate the dangers therein. In order to accomplish this, a shift is required, from the outer focus between the individual and the collective, which is the aim of rites of passage, toward an inner focus, as in the *ukuthwasa* process. The individual with a strengthened ego now strives for a synthesis of consciousness with the unconscious psyche. A new wholeness is constellated between consciousness and the unconscious, and this is not to be mistaken as a regressive movement. As Neumann (1954) elaborated:

The aim underlying the archetype of initiation is for the ego to become conscious of the self. Therefore, this is no longer the hero conquering the dragon, but rather the assimilation with the unconscious content as the conscious mind experiences the unity of the psyche with the resultant shift of the center of the personality from the ego to the self. (pp. 412)

Dangers still threaten the ego on this journey as it is confronted with the multiplicity of the archetype where figures are more complex and less personal and where the phenomenon of the transcendent is activated: the uniting symbol, which is the product of the attitude of the ego in its capacity to face the unconscious (see also chapter 10). This phase is no longer collectively determined, but individual. This initiation does not occur in the collective ceremonial space but is an inner journey for the initiate. The end result of the under the water initiation is not only the safe return, but rather the ability to maintain a particular transpersonal knowledge independent of any human agency. In the resultant transformation, the healer is not just a more effective member of the group. More pertinent, from a psychological perspective, the outcome of the initiation as a whole also separates her from the outer collective, as she is required to serve the personal and the collective unconscious, ego and Self. Ntombi reflected after this experience:

It helps you understand who you are, where you come from, so you know about yourself. My spirit has been healed; my soul was crying out to be recognized, but I did not know how to see the signs. I gained my identity, reconnected with my ancestors, my roots. It gave me better insight into myself and other people. It gave me knowledge and wisdom, and it made me complete. But it was also very lonely. People fear and reject you as you have the knowledge.

Striving for Wholeness

This initiation journey is a quest for individuation, a psychic wholeness in which the ego is subordinate to the Self, and simultaneously in an active relationship with the Self.

Psychologically, the under the water experience can be understood as that which takes place within the retort of the healer's inner world. The impact of this process is said to have both a psychic and a material quality: Both healer and inner psychic energy are transformed.

What Corbin, and later Jung, seemed to know, and what the above account describes, is a movement out of external reality into an inner topography that cannot be found in any cartographer's rendition. Rather this requires a movement beyond the Western mind's tendency toward disbelief, with the resultant dichotomy between logos and Eros. This internalized movement, with the phenomena of spirit in matter, is one that encapsulates the African healing cosmology in its entirety, and one that underlies the understanding of the concept of the ancestors discussed in chapter 2. Jung (1961a) reflected that the "figures of my fantasies brought home to me the crucial insight that there are things in the psyche which I do not produce, but which produce themselves and have their own life" (p. 207). Ntombi came to understand this as a psychological fact underlying her calling within her cultural heritage, and she felt encouraged to embrace her calling. As Ntombi's process reached a culmination, she had the following dream:

> *I am lying dying on my bed at home. I am dressed in white and my face is painted with white clay. A man dressed as a healer comes to me and gives me the red clay face paint, red and white ceremonial beads, a new animal skin and healing regalia. He insists that I go with him. I resist, but he remains adamant. We fly together and he shows me where to find and how to prepare healing herbs that I must use for my healing and those I must use for others who are ill. Then I see myself dressed in my multicolored regalia, many, many colors all woven into one.*

This dream brought comfort to Ntombi on her path to healing. In the dream she is shown where to find healing by an ancestral figure. The flying figure evokes the winged Mercurius, a guide between the conscious and unconscious, a psychopomp and an intermediary between the suffering initiate and an experience of death. Similarly, in the Greek myth, Hermes guides the soul through times of transition and symbolizes that aspect capable of moving between opposites. Von Franz (1986) described the flying figure in death dreams as "a still unknown aspect of [the dreamer's] soul [which] comes to the dying dreamer in order to conduct her to the other side" (p. 73). For the healer, this symbolizes the capacity to move, at will, into the transpersonal.

The dream also reflects the need for the old to die in order for the new to emerge. The images of Ntombi lying dying on her bed and then flying seem symbolic of a death and of the transitional space that requires the temporary "setting aside" of the ego position. This dream seems to present another image of the enantiodromia with respect to the *nigredo* and the underwater account described above. Here, Ntombi ascends into the heavens, countering her descent into the depths of the unconscious waters.

Ntombi is required to find the right *muthi* for her own healing. She is required to ceremoniously embrace her calling and adorn herself with the traditional markings in the form of the red and white beads, a new skin, and the full color range of her healer's apparel. In so doing, she heals herself and learns the healing practices of how to heal others in turn. It is in this dream

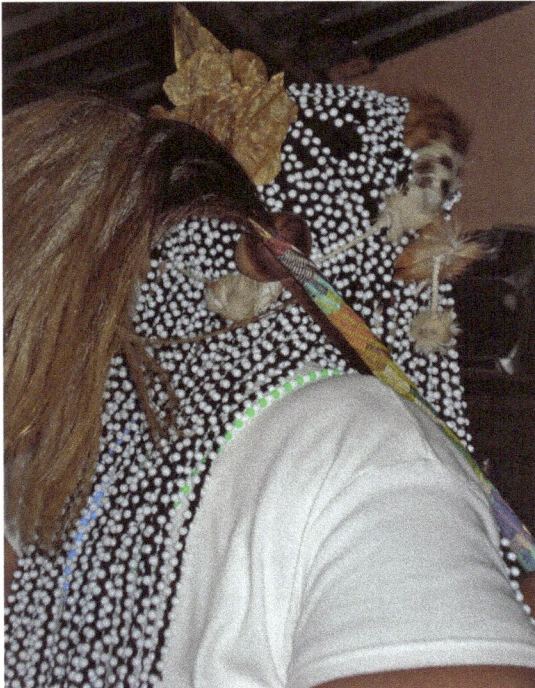

Figure 36. White beads of a healer's headpiece

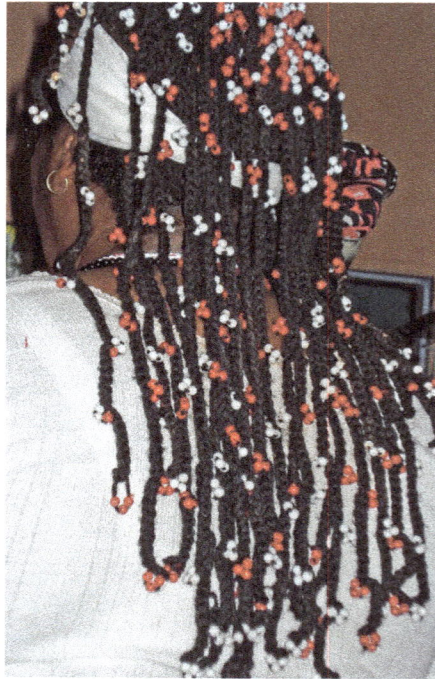

Figure 37. The combination of red and white beads in the regalia of a healer

that an image of the fully evolved healer, with the combination of the red and white finally emerges.

For the African healer, the white beads symbolize the feminine in that they represent the ancestral spirits of the maternal line. The red beads are indicative of the paternal line. The theme of the white and red in the clothes, face paint, beads, and *muthi* parallel the alchemical symbolism of the pair of opposites, the basic polarity between masculine and feminine principles.

It is with the final stage of the initiation that the red and white beads are combined, symbolic of a union of opposites. This combination symbolizes the initiate's proficiency with opposite energies contained within the paternal and maternal lines. Psychologically, the feminine and masculine principles are awakened. Both are considered necessary for ultimate physical and psychic health as well as for optimum functioning of the healer. The alchemical image of the red and white rose, the "golden flower" of alchemy, symbolic of the birthplace of the *filius philosophorum,* or *lapis*, the end result of the opus can be juxtaposed here (see Jung, 1944, p.77).

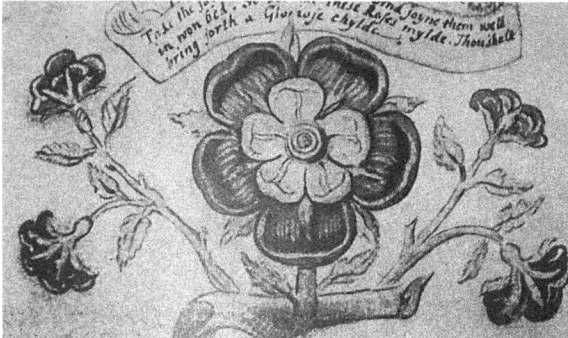

Figure 38. The red and white rose, the "golden flower" of alchemy,
as the birthplace of the *filius philosophorum*

The Alchemical *Coniunctio*

An outcome of both the alchemical opus and the African healing initiation is the bridging of the divide between opposites. There is a coming together of two aspects and the emergence of something new, as embodied in the meaning of the word *ukuthwasa*, discussed in chapter 4. For the initiate, the *coniunctio* of the initiation process is an open channel to the ancestral voices, and psychologically, a bringing together of ego consciousness with the unconscious, the inner with the outer. Edinger (1991) commented on the outcome with respect to the alchemical opus:

> The *coniunctio* is the culmination of the opus . . . it has both an extraverted and introverted aspect. The alchemists' fascination with the *coniunctio* on the extraverted side prompted a study of the miracle of chemical combination and led to modern chemistry and nuclear physics. On the introverted side it generated interest in unconscious imagery and processes, leading to twentieth-century depth psychology. (p. 211)

In a similar fashion, the healer's role embodies both the internal and the external. Externally, the healer develops a capacity to heal and an intimate knowledge of the herbal remedies. This includes the preparation of the herbs and the use thereof for various ailments. Not unlike the alchemist in his laboratory, the healers grow and cultivate their own pharmacopoeia of indigenous herbs and subject the herbs to various

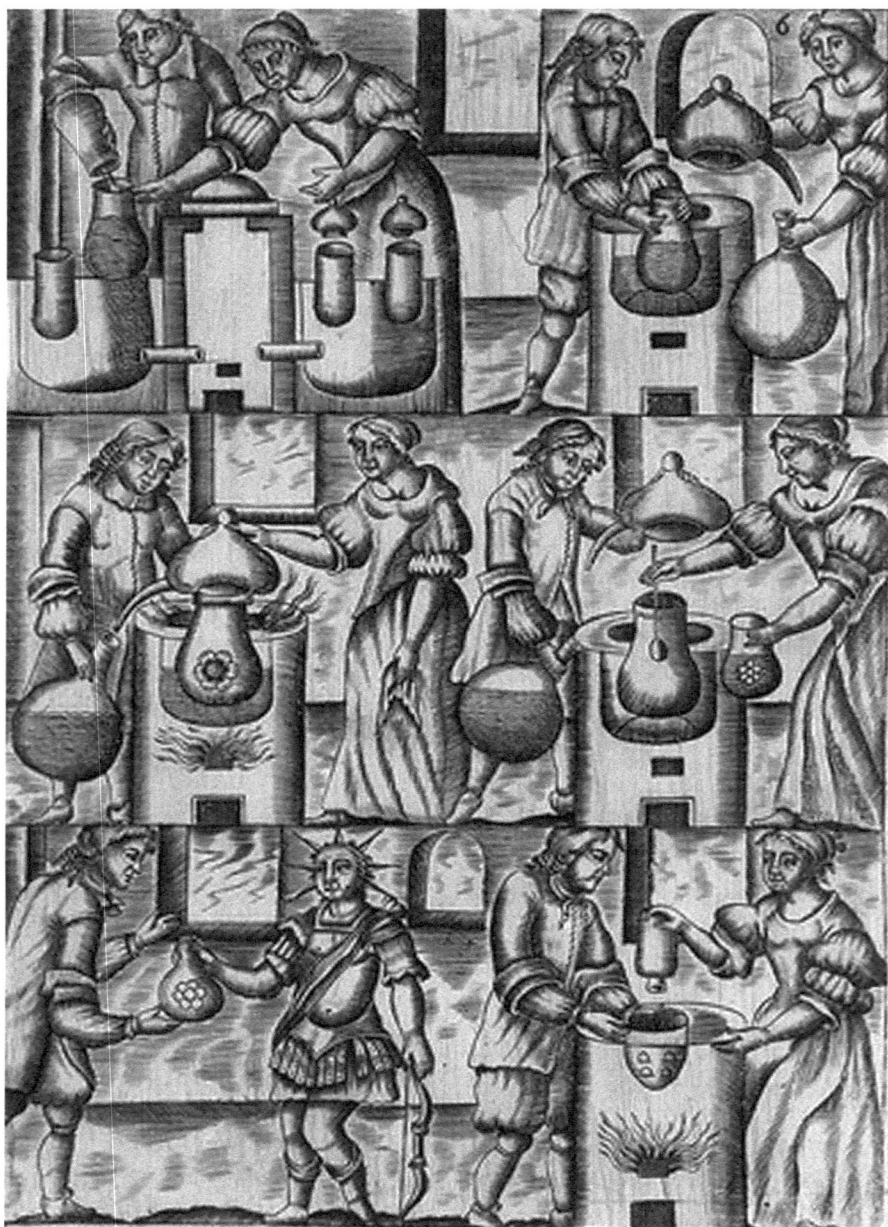

Figure 39. The stages of the alchemical process with the alchemists at work depicting the various stages of transformation of the golden flower as symbolic of the Self within the alchemical retort. Mutus Liber, pl. 6

chemical transformations through burning, dissolving, and imbibing these remedies. The pharmacological effects of these herbs are only now being subjected to rigorous, so-called scientific, evidence-based research. Results confirm what the healers have always known: the chemical and pharmaceutical healing properties of the herbs (Radomsky, 2006, p. 477).

On the inner level, the initiate develops an open living vein to the unconscious, the transpersonal, with the focus on ancestral communications and dream symbolism. As such, creative and respectful acknowledgment of the autonomy of the unconscious emerges, which mirrors the relationship nurtured by the depth psychologist.

The *coniunctio*, in the alchemical opus, is often symbolized by an image of marriage. Jung, in a discussion on the components of the *coniunctio* and the personification of opposites, explained that the corresponding masculine substance is the red sulphur, the *servus rubeus* (red slave) or *servus rubicundus* (1955–56, para. 16, n. 105). The feminine substance is the *femina candida* or *femina alba* (white woman), or white substance. This symbolism is embedded in the combination of the red and the white beads of the healer. Jung explained that after the *rubedo*, there is an increase in consciousness and a "synthesis of opposites . . . in which the marriage of the red man and the white woman, or opposites Sol and Luna, is consummated" (1955–56, para. 307). The image of marriage is an image of the union of opposites, the *coniunctio*, the *hieros gamos* or mystical marriage found throughout many mythological, psychological, and alchemical texts: Tiferet and Shekhinah of the Jewish Kabbalists; the union of Israel and the God of the Hebrews in the Song of Songs; Zeus and Hera in the Greek pantheon; Sol and Luna in the alchemical opus; the crucifixion; yin and yang, the cosmic principles; psyche and matter, to mention a few. Ntombi described her understanding:

It is about spirituality. It is the maternal earth part or the paternal spirit part that makes a person ill. Too much male energy or too much female energy in a person makes them ill. Both sides need to be strong and in balance. We must discover which side is lacking and that is the side that must be strengthened.

The union of opposites referred to here with respect to the outcome of the initiation process is the healer's ability to harness, at will, the healing

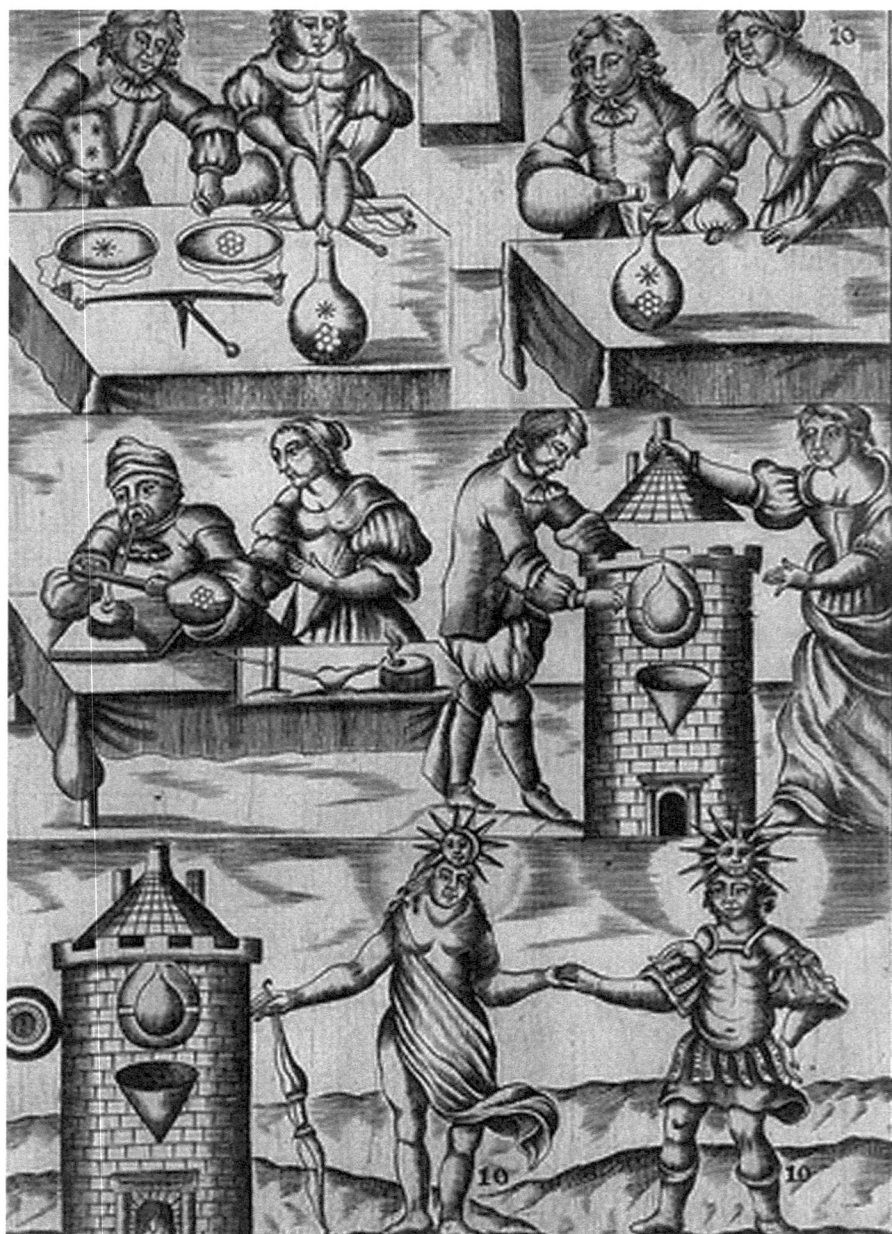

Figure 40. Alchemists at work: the upper two thirds showing the stages of the process and the lower third the *coniunctio* of opposites symbolized by the male and female pair. Mutus liber, pl. 10

forces carried by the ancestors. The initiate, as symbolic of the *prima materia*, through the initiation rituals, is subjected to what the alchemists described in the preparation of the stone. Commenting on the emergence of the *coniunctio*, Edinger (1991) explained that

> the goal of the opus is the creation of a miraculous entity variously called the Philosopher's Stone . . . It is produced by the final union of purified opposites, and because it combines the opposites, it mitigates and rectifies all one sidedness. (p. 215)

According to the alchemists, the stone has the power to transform the *prima materia*, or the base matter, into that of the supreme value. Once activated, this ability of the stone seems to have a living quality in that its effect multiplies, like cells dividing; it grows and augments. As the stone is a symbol or an image of the Self, the implication here is that the Self carries this capacity. As Edinger (1991) explained, this embodies the alchemical operation of the *multiplicatio* and "suggests that transformative effects emanate from the activated self in the process of conscious realization" (p. 227). As such, an individual in conscious relationship to the Self seems to have the capacity to infect others with a germ of consciousness. One can see this in psychobiographical and historical accounts of great personalities who have the ability to affect others and to transform attitudes, Nelson Mandela being a local and global example of this phenomenon.

Ntombi's development in the analytical retort as well as her progress in the initiatory realm was anticipated by the following dream:

> *I'm getting married. The setting is a beautiful ancient stone enclosure. The novice healers are helping me to dress. I have been fasting for three days. They bathe me and rub my skin with fragrant oils. They bring my bridal regalia to dress me. It's a deep crimson color, sewn with silk and patterned with intricate multi-colored beads. It feels like a second skin. In the centre of the dress is a circular silvery-white pattern embroidered into the material. The healers lead me out to where the wedding ceremony will take place. Standing waiting to receive me is the groom. I have a deep sense of peace.*

At the same time, I had the following dream:

I am in an old garden that has a feeling of timelessness. In the centre of the garden is a large natural body of water. A huge ancient tree stands in the centre of the water. Its branches reach out to the circumference of the lake, which is filled with bird life. One bird emerges from the flock. It is large, a deep violet color with blue and green crested feathers. I watch as the bird nests under the tree.

Cauda Pavonis: The Peacock's Tail

As the *thwasa* reaches the completion of her initiation and training, the regalia can take on very individual and quite colorful appearance.[18] Each initiate is said to dream of what the final regalia will look like. The details are communicated to the senior healer, who prepares the regalia according to the dream. At this time, the uniqueness of the healer emerges. Here we are reminded of the end of the alchemical process (or at times the beginning) whereby the material of the stone causes beautiful colors to appear. Jung (1942) amplified these colors to suggest the many colors of the *cauda pavonis.* The appearance of the peacock's tail variously heralds the transition out of the darkness of the *nigredo,* as well as the immanent attainment of the goal (para. 190, n. 90).

Jung explained that the many colors that emerge after the *nigredo,* through the *albedo* and *rubedo* are latent in the *nigredo* (1946b, para. 479–480). Here Jung likens the *nigredo* to the flooding of the Nile; in other words, the dark earth contains within it the fertility for a new birth. The *nigredo* thus exists as the necessary precursor to new life. The image of the *cauda pavonis* and the appearance of the colors in the alchemical vessel, like the multicolored regalia of the healer, denote the spring and the renewal of life: a *post tenebras lux.* As Jung (1955-56) elucidates:

The *cauda pavonis* is also called the "soul of the world, nature, the quintessence, which causes all things to bring forth." Here the peacock occupies the highest place as a symbol . . . in whom the male-female polarity . . . is integrated. (para. 392)

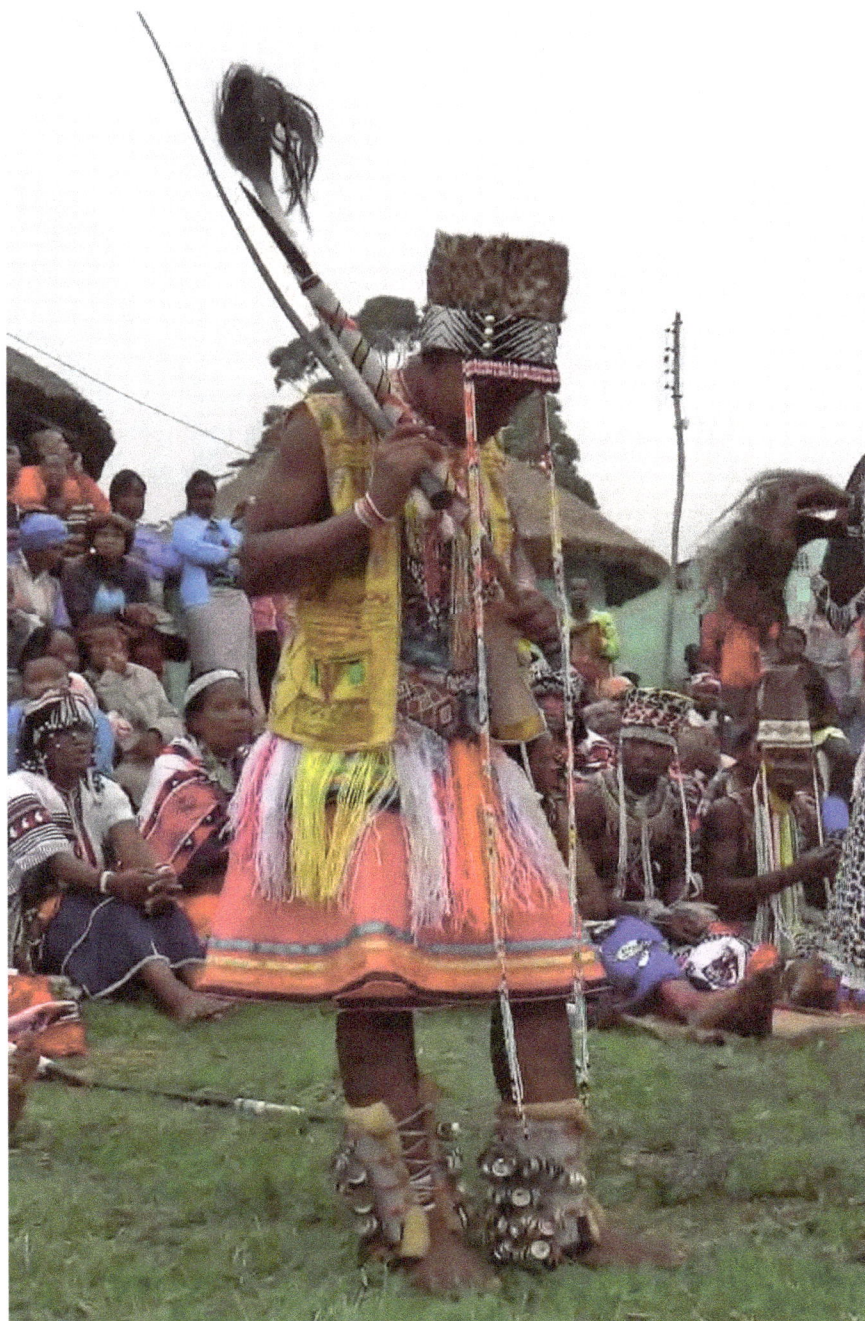

Figure 41. A healer displays her multicolored regalia at her graduation ceremony

And further:

> The *cauda pavonis* announces the end of the work . . . The exquisite display of colors in the peacock's fan heralds the imminent synthesis of all qualities and elements, which are united in the "rotundity" of the philosophical stone. (para. 397)

The peacock can further be amplified as a bird of immortality with the "eyes" in the tail feathers suggesting the capacity of all-seeing eternal vision. In early Christian symbolism the peacock signified resurrection, rebirth, and eternal life. The image of resurrection connects the peacock to the Christian symbol of the savior and the phoenix, born anew from the ashes. Von Franz (1980a) explained that "the peacock, symbolising the renewal of life, rises from the sealed retort . . . in which takes place the union of opposites, the integration of masculine and feminine" (p. 158).

Psychologically, this play of color heralds the return of life after a state of death, a state that is experienced by the *thwasa*, who from the initial *nigredo* through to the *albedo* and *rubedo* has existed without a full identity. The changing of the colors in the healer's regalia symbolizes psychologically the stages of transition. Jung (1955–56) explained that the display of colors "means that during the assimilation of the unconscious the personality passes through many transformations, which show in different lights and are followed by ever changing moods. These changes presage the coming birth" (para. 430).

Here, once again, the symbol of the indomitable spirit Mercurius seems relevant. Both in the alchemical opus and in the realm of the African healer, the symbol of Mercurius seems to capture that elusive indefinable something that is the healing or the "gold" in the stone. Jung summarized the numerous aspects of Mercurius to include all conceivable opposites and "as such, he represents on the one hand the self and on the other the individuation process and . . . also the collective unconscious" (1948g, para. 284). Jung (1944) explained that when

> the alchemist speaks of Mercurius, on the face of it he means quicksilver, but inwardly he means the world-creating spirit concealed or imprisoned in matter. . . . Mercurius stands at the beginning and the end of the work: he is the *prima materia* . . .

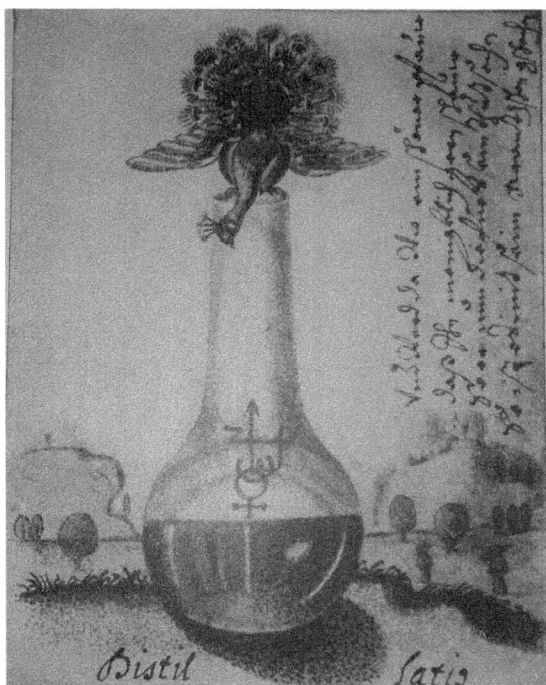

Figure 42: Peacock symbolizing the renewal of life,
rising from the sealed retort

the *nigredo* . . . He is the play of colors in the *cauda pavonis* and the division into four elements . . . and is reunited in the *coniunctio*, to appear once again at the end in the radiant form of the *lumen novum*, the stone. He is metallic yet liquid, matter yet spirit, cold yet fiery, poison and yet healing draught—a symbol uniting all opposites. (para. 404)

In her dream, Ntombi sees her multicolored apparel, and she is required to accept a "new skin," symbolic of her acceptance of the calling back to the Self. Ntombi's new skin seemed to constellate the emergence of a new image of the Self, no longer a projected Self or an imitation, no longer the oppressed black self-image nor the identification with white oppressor self-image.

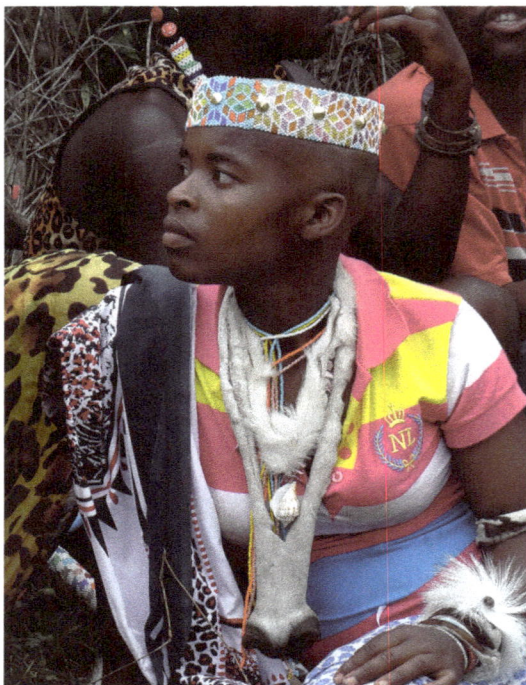

Figure 43. A healer at her graduation ceremony with the multicolored headpiece design that she had seen in a dream

At this point, the initiate is once again concealed in a hut for a period of isolation. After a time of deep introversion and meditation during her seclusion, she is only seen again when she reappears, dressed in her full glory to the celebratory welcome of the community of healers. This is a momentous occasion, pregnant with numinous energy and expectation, quite literally the birth of the healer. It is deeply moving to be present at the moment when the sealed hut is opened and to witness the emergence of the healer, radiant in her full regalia. The appearance of the fully developed healer after the final seclusion seems to reflect the aspect of a renewal and an image of the union of opposites.

Chapter 10
Unio Mystica:
As Above, So Below

There is a world beyond ours—a world where everything is known.
—Ntombi

As our work progressed, Ntombi was able to reflect more deeply on her conflict around her repulsion of the inner forces of her ancestral life and her identification with Western ways. She had fought for what she had perceived to be her only hope, that of adopting Western beliefs, of becoming "white." In so doing, she was caught in a complex that had resulted in her rejection of her natural way of being.

I had begun to understand Ntombi's crisis on a deeper archetypal level as her rejection of the urge from the Self to incarnate in her as an authentic experience. I came to see her struggle as an embodiment of the attempt to integrate deeper levels of the unconscious through the reconciliation of opposites. This had manifested in her ego's protection against a loss of autonomy as she feared that she would be controlled by forces within her. She had resisted the calling from the Self to reawaken her personal numinosity. As such, she had suffered a loss of soul, a severing of her relationship with her inner psychic life.

For Ntombi, her conflict seemed to reside in her ego's one-sided attitude to the Self, and she was called to forsake this in order for the new to emerge. She was faced with a crisis that seemed to offer no rational solution and that would require the birth of the irrational "other." Marie-Louise von Franz (1997a) reflected that this is an expression of the objective psyche in that the unconscious seems to be seeking a realization of something new that has never been there before, something creatively new, yet something new that does not do away with the old but rather adds something to it.

Indigenous cosmologies understand that physical and psychic symptoms are often symbols of a soul sickness: a disconnection from the spirit, the symbol, the myth and ritual, with the resultant loss of the ancestral balance and loss of meaning in life. For indigenous cultures, in order to correct a dysfunctional state, whether physical or psychic, there is a need to first locate the hidden symbolic dimension through the ritual.

This process mirrors Jung's concept of symbol formation as a synthetic reconstruction of the symbol and not just a reduction to the natural condition. Jung (1948a) conceived of ritual as a gradient for the libido and noted:

> The enormous complexity of such ceremonies shows how much is needed to divert the libido from its natural river bed of everyday habit into some unaccustomed activity. The modern mind thinks this can be done by a mere decision of will and it can dispense with all magical ceremonies. . . . Through these ceremonies the deeper emotional forces are released . . . on which the whole weight of the unconscious forces is concentrated. (para. 87)

For Ntombi, this complexity required letting go of the idea that all can be known and embracing the epistemology of the healer as one in which body, mind, and spirit all belong together. In Jung's (1951) words:

> Psyche and matter exist in one and the same world, and each partakes of the other, otherwise any reciprocal action would be impossible. If research could only advance far enough, therefore, we should arrive at an ultimate agreement between physical and psychological concepts. (para. 413)

With the loss of everything to which she had attached value, Ntombi was plunged into a state of despair and alienation. Psychologically, for her, the *ukuthwasa* initiation represented the experience of something unintentional, something strange, and something objective, which reflected Jung's (1997) comment of "the experience of something which is not I, yet is still psychical" (p. 73).

A further loss for Ntombi was the loss of religious projection, which in turn often constellates a confrontation with the Self. She was offered the

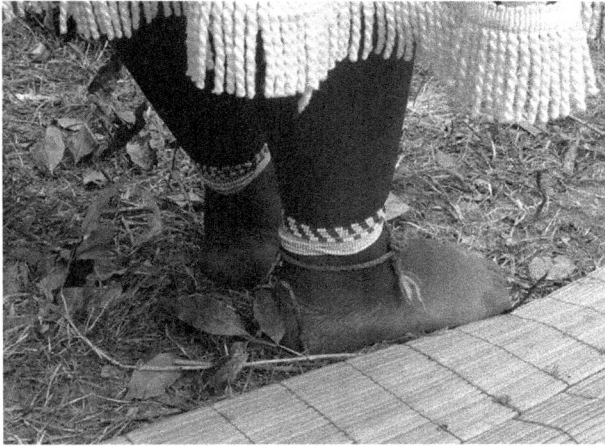

Figure 44: Ankle beads worn by the healers

opportunity to face the ultimate questions in life, and she was able to use this opportunity for a decisive development in consciousness. What was required of her, in her awareness of her despair and isolation, was a growing awareness of her distinctiveness, which resulted in a tension of opposites that provided the stimulation for further consciousness. She was called to confront her early childhood identity through the activation of the unconscious in the *ukuthwasa* initiation. For Ntombi, the adopted collective religion of her parents had become inadequate, and she was called to divest herself of the collective beliefs of the white religious dogma. The effect of her unconscious identification with the white oppressor, growing up praying to the white God-image, had resulted in Ntombi's rejection of her ancestral communications and the language of her soul.

The Evolving God-Image

Ntombi's initiation into the African healing paradigm, as well as her analysis in the analytical context, offered her an entry into an inner experience that manifests in what could be considered, for her, a new God-image. Edinger (1996) elucidates that "individuation, the discovery of the psyche, refers to the psychological level which understands religious imagery as the phenomenology of the objective psyche" (p. xxi). According to Jung (1951), the God-image holds "the highest value and supreme dominant in the psychic hierarchy . . . immediately related to, or identical with, the self" (para. 170). This seemed to embody Ntombi's conflict at the beginning of her process, and in this way the loss of her early religious projection served a salutary purpose: It became the stimulus that led to the development of an individual personality. Jung (1937) explained:

> The ultimate cause of a neurosis is something *positive* which needs to be safeguarded for the patient; otherwise he suffers a psychic loss. . . . The childhood experience of the neurotic is not, in itself, negative. . . . It becomes negative only when it finds no suitable place in the life and the outlook of the adult. The real task of analysis . . . is to bring about a synthesis between the two. (para. 564)

I reflected on Jung's (1943) idea of the transcendent function, a symbol or image that often emerges in dreams during periods of conflict or transition, capable of transcending consciousness, and the conflict of opposites, or one-sidedness. That is, the transcendent has a teleological function that strives for a union of opposites. Ntombi's process appeared to be indicative of the emergence of the transcendent function, defined as that which facilitates a transition from one attitude to another, wherein opposites potentially encounter each other (Samuels, Shorter, & Plaut, 1991). Jung (1958) elaborated that it is the transcendent function, the symbol forming spirit, which makes the transition from a one-sided attitude to a new and more complete one organically possible (para. 137).

This epitomized Ntombi's despair where she had embraced the Western paradigm and was being held for ransom by a numinous other. She was faced with the eternal struggle of a relativistic reality against an irrational force that haunted her dreams. The force manifested as her "illness," and in its resolution, it would prepare her to be a healer.

Otto (1958) defined numinous as that which displaces our will with its own. Jung (1951) observed that the numinous is potentially overwhelming and that perhaps the ego's refusal to begin dialogue with invisible forces is a protection against that which might seem to threaten the conscious mind. For Ntombi, these "invisible forces" held a certain objective reality as they represented the ancestors.

For Ntombi to *see* her blackness meant confronting all the projections of the white culture that she had unconsciously accepted. Her identification of black as negative had resulted in the rejection of her core being, in a desperate attempt to become the other. In this she could only but fail.

During the *ukuthwasa* process, the ego consciously encounters a link to a divine agency in the form of the ancestors that supports, commands, or directs, and which psychologically, we can understand as the ego's encounter with the Self. As Jung (1951) discovered, the Self needs conscious realization and is obliged by the individuation urge to tempt and test the ego in order to bring about full ego awareness of the existence of the Self. *Ukuthwasa,* psychologically, is a breakup of the conscious status quo by an influx of fiery energy from the unconscious that divests the initiate of the persona. Such an image heralds an individuation crisis, with the potential for a major step in the psychological development.

The task of the individual, thus Ntombi's task, as noted by Edinger (1972), is to develop a wider consciousness and to divest the Self of the false wrappings of the persona. In so doing, each individual is imbued with the capability of transforming the collective unconscious God-image. Von Franz (1997a) elaborated that whenever the archetypal layers are activated in an individual, it can become either a source of creative restructuring and new spiritual realizations or, if something goes wrong, it can become a source of pathological states and actions.

Through the *ukuthwasa* initiation, a conscious attitude of submission to the process of transformation is encouraged. This entails the ego's recognition of the transpersonal other and its own subordinate position, as well as its preparedness to serve the totality, even if this goes counter to conscious personal desires. Ntombi came to recognize that by embracing her ancestral forces, she gained a freedom not previously conceived of, and that it was her very denial of them that kept her imprisoned in her conflict, unable to realize her potential.

This mirrors what can happen psychologically, that true meaning lies in what had appeared to be rejected, and what was considered to be error is revealed to be full of significance, wherein the irrational finds acceptance. Ntombi's dreams, particularly of the distorted animals and the calling into her cultural origins, confronted her with an overwhelming tension. Her conscious belief system was challenged, and this resulted in an inner split that would be healed only to the extent that she could embrace a more authentic connection with the Self. As Jung (1946b) outlined:

> The painful conflict that begins with the *nigredo* . . . described by the alchemists . . . as dismemberment of the body, excruciating animal sacrifices. . . . While this extreme form of *disiunctio* is going on, there is a transformation of that arcanum—be it substance or spirit—which invariably turns out to be the mysterious Mercurius. In other words, out of the monstrous animal forms there gradually emerges a *res simplex,* whose nature is one and the same and yet consists of a duality. . . . His gold is *non vulgi*, his *lapis* is spirit and body, and so is his tincture, which is a *sanguis spiritualis*—a spiritual blood. (para. 398)

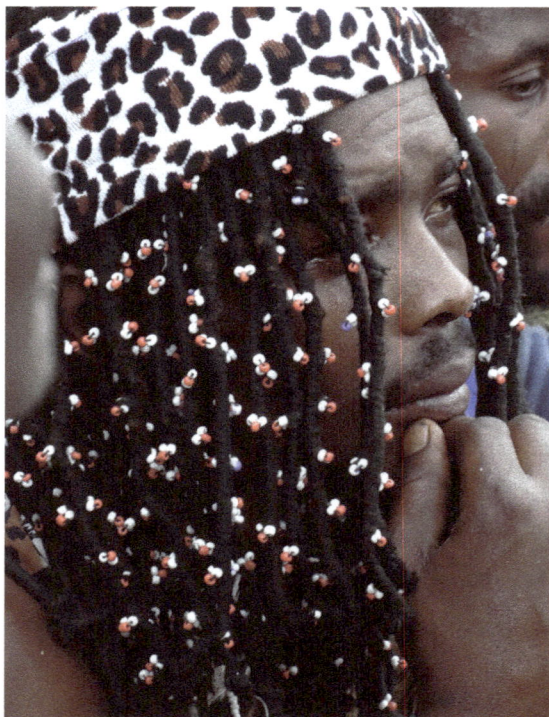

Figure 45. A senior male healer, Eastern Cape, South Africa

The African healer has a rapport with nature and its transcendental energies, which guide and support. The initiation experience embodies a creative living psychological relationship to the inner world. Ntombi had arrived at the beginning of her analysis in a state of anguish. Her distress appeared to be a manifestation of the divine conflict, wherein she was caught between her distorted adopted identity and that of her calling to honor the Self within her cultural matrix. She seemed to embody the confusion often experienced when there is an encounter with the Self or the paradoxical nature of God. Jung (1952a) explained that such an encounter bears the risk for the individual in that it potentially "tears man asunder into opposites and delivers him over to a seemingly insoluble conflict" (para. 738).

The initiation in the *ukuthwasa* vessel and in the analytical retort offered Ntombi a path along which to navigate her personal neurotic conflict and to nurture her relationship with the objective psyche. Psychologically, the individuation urge, related to in a conscious way, potentially promotes a state in which the ego is related to the Self without being identified with it. Out of this state, there emerges a more or less continuous dialogue between the conscious ego and the unconscious, between inner and outer experience. The elements of the African healing initiation, as described, contain the ingredients for a dialogue between the ego and the Self via the ancestors and toward a reconciliation of opposites and the emergence of a new personal myth. Edinger (1984) commented that "the new myth tells us that each individual ego is the crucible for the creation of consciousness and a vessel to serve as a carrier of that consciousness" (p. 32).

Ntombi was faced with the reality of a deep inner source and center of psychic life with its own sense of purposefulness. She was faced with an initiation into a new world of profound numinosity. As such, the healer's journey is akin to the alchemical quest whereby the neurotic symptom born out of chaos, and the *ukuthwasa* illness, or the unpleasant rejected *prima materia*, holds the hidden gold. Jung noted (1946b) that

the difficulties of the psychotherapeutic work teach us to take truth, goodness and beauty where we find them. They are not always found where we look for them: often they are hidden in the dirt, or are in the keeping of the dragon. *"In stercore invenitur"* (it is found in the filth) runs an alchemical dictum. (para. 384)

As C.A. Meier (1984) succinctly recorded, "the healer is able to heal because of his own sickness" (p. 24). Thus the process of the initiation is reflective of the ancient myth of the wounded healer in the tradition of Chiron, Asclepius, Galen, Epidaurus, and Pergamum of ancient Greece. Here, illness is seen as the result of divine intervention (or I would say interference) and is only healed by divine intervention. The healer is thus both the illness and its remedy.

As such, Ntombi, as an individual engaged in the inner transformative process, arrived at a more integrated identity, symbolized by a potential realization of her role in the evolution of the inner God-image. This included the realization of the reality of the psyche, which was Jung's ultimate aim. It meant the possibility of embracing both the light and the dark aspects of the Self and a resultant meaningful relationship to her life. As Jung (1951) stressed

transformations in the God-image which run parallel with changes in human consciousness. . . . The God-image is not something *invented*, it is an *experience* that comes upon man spontaneously . . . The unconscious God-image can therefore alter the state of consciousness, just as the latter can modify the God-image once it has become conscious. (para. 303)

The analysis of Ntombi accompanied her initiation into the realm of the African healer by supporting the development of an enlivened and vitalized relationship to and with the unconscious. During this time, Ntombi came to trust and value the inner logic of the unconscious, its creative function in the form of spontaneous images and symbols that often emerge during times of deep despair.

This emergence of unconscious material resulted in a shift from her rational and reductive conscious attitude toward a glimpse of the archetypal layer underlying the symbols and images of the African healing initiation journey. This, in turn, provided a rich backdrop for the unfolding of an individuation process. Jung (1975) explained:

The whole course of individuation is dialectical, and the so-called "end" is the confrontation of the ego with the "emptiness" of the center. . . . In the individuation process the ego is brought face to face with an unknown superior power. (pp. 259-260)

By "emptiness" Jung was referring to something "unknowable." For Ntombi, the nascent outcome of this shift was the change in the relationship between ego and Self, with the awareness of the transpersonal archetypal forces embedded in her cultural heritage. This awareness had been lost to her consciousness due to a number of external challenges. At a crisis point in her life, she found herself faced with a new emerging pattern that required an adjustment to inner forces, the world of inner images, which, in order to access, required a relationship with the unconscious.

Psychologically, she was faced with an internal polarization, a deep unconscious inner split that manifested in an excess of adaptation. Her vehement and often self-destructive denial of her calling back to her cultural and spiritual heritage reflected her biographical life experiences of poverty, oppression, and inferiority. She had lived out a pattern of a collective psychology in identification with collective values. Her conscious adaptation and conscious attitude had reached its limits and had become too narrow, which resulted in a conflict. Conflict is often the precondition for the stimulation of symbol formation, and if successfully negotiated, can lead to reconciliation.

While working with Ntombi, I was given a fleeting glimpse of the religious function of the psyche, in that the religious function aims to link the ego back to its origins as well as to give careful consideration to the source of one's being. The African healing cosmology seems to encapsulate a living experience of the connection to a greater whole. Pivotal to this relationship is the phenomenon of the ancestors, the living dead.

The Living Dead Revisited

Throughout the ages, the idea has existed that after death something endures or is continuous. This seems to be in accord with a psychological understanding, as von Franz (1987) noted, that "the unconscious believes quite obviously in a life after death" (p. xi.). This concept, expressed through various symbols, captures an aspect of the phenomenon that the soul possesses a kind of subtle body. This is embodied in the alchemist's concepts of *meditatio* and *imaginatio* and bears a similarity to the relationship of the healer to the ancestors.

For the alchemists, the *meditatio* implied an inner dialogue or a living relationship to the "other" within, psychologically, the unconscious. Jung (1944), in citing the alchemist Ruland, identified the term *imaginatio* as central to the alchemical opus as "the star in man, the celestial or supercelestial body" (para. 394). Jung continued, noting that the *imaginatio* must be conceived of not just as an act of fantasy, but as "producing something more corporeal, a 'subtle body,' semi-physical in nature" (1944, para. 394). This concept is as central to understanding the African healing realm as it was to the alchemical opus. As Jung (1944) expounded with respect to the alchemistic ways of thought wherein there existed

> an intermediate realm between mind and matter, i.e., a psychic realm of subtle bodies whose characteristic it is to manifest themselves in a mental as well as a material form . . . and the physical and the psychic are once more blended in an indissoluble unity. (para. 394)

This is an expression of an archetypal idea, carefully articulated by von Franz in her book *On Dreams and Death* (1987). In antiquity, as noted by von Franz, Pythagoreans and Platonists spoke of a radiating subtle body. Plato describes the soul as encompassed in brightness. Neo-Platonists refer to a "light soul," a starlike eternal light. Plutarch, in the second century, described the soul's continuous color as surrounded by a flame-like covering, some with continuous color, some with discolorations and slight scratches.

The concept of the subtle body is a complex one that defies definition and remains a mystery. It is a phenomenon that can only be glimpsed in experiences. It can be understood, in psychological terms, as that which is has been incorporated into consciousness from the unconscious. In other words, an aspect of the unconscious *prima materia* that has been purified and is now accessible to consciousness, but which differs from ego consciousness in that it is a materialized aspect of spirit, that is, a manifestation of unconscious psychic energy within the imagination that has a psychological reality and a quality of being. In short, the idea of subtle bodies is related to the understanding that there is a link between pure spirit and material body, and in my view, helps us to grasp an aspect of the phenomenon of the living dead. Here again, Jung (1948e) assists with this phenomenon when he explained:

Our world of consciousness and the "Beyond" together form a single cosmos, with the result that the dead are not in a different place from the living. There is only a difference in their "frequencies," . . . where the unconscious possesses a higher energy. (para. 752)

The unity of the here and there is a familiar concept in the African healer's life. Both coexist in continual ongoing interaction, each influencing the other: the material world and the ancestral world, the realm of the living dead. The healer moves into the ancestral world and has an effect on it. In a reciprocal fashion, the living dead or the ancestors have an effect on the living, material world. What exactly it is, we cannot fully know, but for the African healers, that it exists, is an accepted phenomenon, understood and honored in the concept of the ancestors. As noted by Jung (1977):

We are not in the position to prove that anything of us is necessarily preserved for eternity. But we can assume with great probability that something of our psyches goes on existing. . . . In general one could say that since consciousness is an important psychic phenomenon, why shouldn't it be just that part of the psyche which not affected by space and time? In other words it goes on existing relatively outside of space and time . . . an existence for an indefinite time after or beyond death. (pp. 380–381)

The African healer's reverence of life after death seems at times to supersede life, or certainly that life is the preparation for death. Many rituals and ceremonies celebrate death, invite death (in the form of the ancestors) to participate actively in life. This tradition offers what Jung (1961a) advised when he stated "do your best to form a conception of life after death, to create some image of it" (p. 330).

Understanding the phenomenon of the communication with the ancestors, the realm where the soul and the body meet, evokes the concepts of the *coincidentia oppositorum* and the *unus mundus*. Jung (1973) suggested that "in the deepest layers of the unconscious which seem to be spaceless and timeless, there is a relative eternity and a relative non-separation" (p. 257). For Jung, contact with this world of the *unus mundus*

179

is vital for man, and the whole challenge of individuation is to be in its service, that is, to be consciously related to something infinite. Von Franz (1992) explained that the alchemist worked to uncover the original animating spirit of the world, the *unus mundus,* the thought of God (p. 40).

For the healer, the ancestors are a reality. They possess a living ontological status outside of any personal mind. They are experienced during the *ukuthwasa* period that is characterized by submergence in the inner world of dreams and altered states of consciousness. Psychologically, we can understand this as the inclination toward the integration of the unconscious material into consciousness.

The healer has the ability to transverse, at will, the inner numinous realms in order to gain greater knowledge. He or she then returns and presents this new knowledge to the community, and in so doing enhances the connection between the ancestral and physical or human realm. Similarly, the spirit guides of the healer prompt and cajole the individual toward greater awareness and ability. Herein rests the idea of initiation as an image of the individuation process. According to Jung (1954a), individuation involves a circumambulation of the Self, the origin of psychic development as well as the engine of integration and wholeness (para. 341). Ntombi described her awareness of the process as

> listening to the inner man. . . . There is a world beyond ours, what we know, and a world that is far away and nearby, visible and invisible. A world where everything has already happened and everything is known; that world talks to us, it has a language of its own.

A crucial distinction that needs to be highlighted is the differentiation between the phenomenon of spirits of the dead, as noted by von Franz (1974) as "personifications of unconscious contents in the living *or* as real apparitions of the dead themselves" (p. 265, italics added). Jung remained noncommittal despite experiences in his own life, and von Franz stated that this matter had not been clarified. In my experience as well as numerous experiences that I have collected from healers, the reality of both phenomena emerges. During the initiation, the initiate is introduced to the ancestral spirits who become guides in the healing process. How exactly this unfolds once again must remain a mystery, however, the phenomenon that

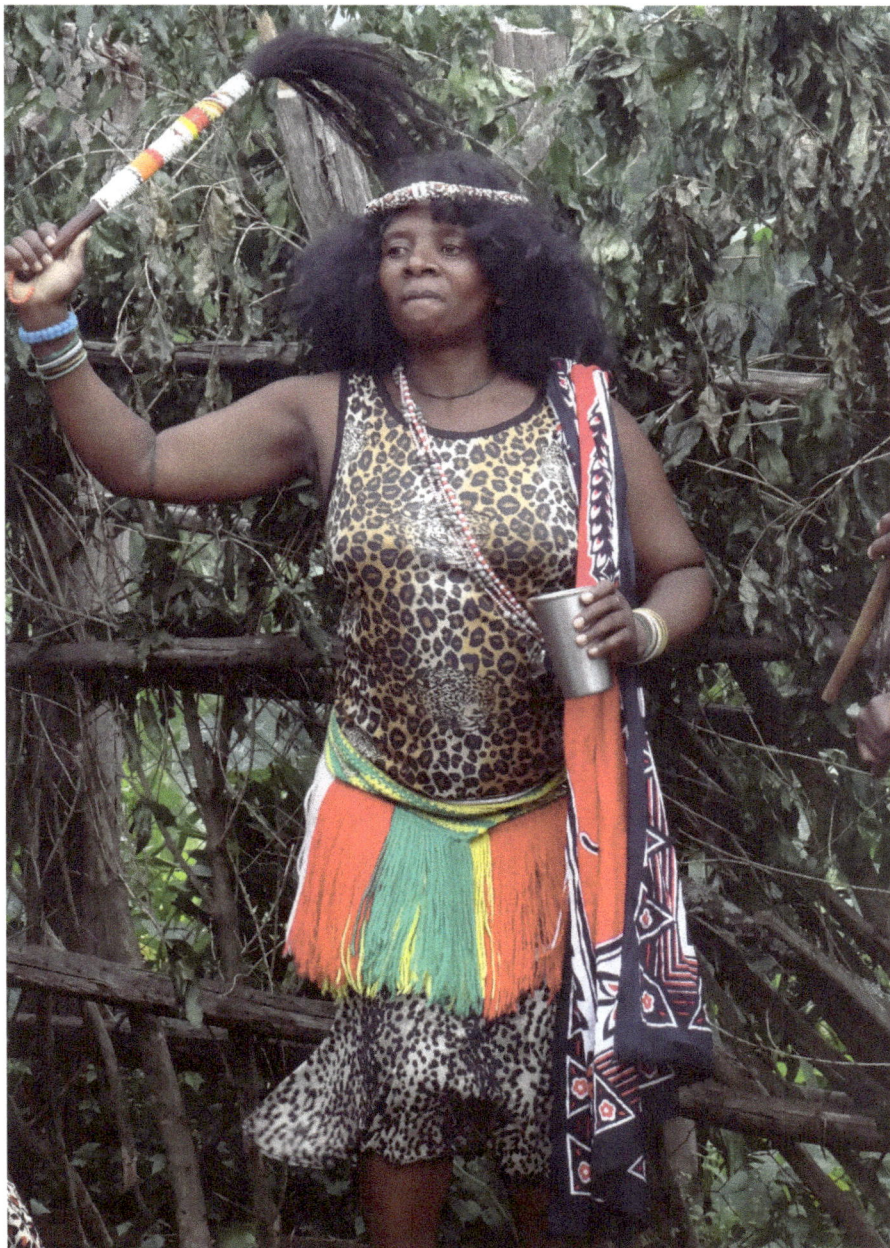

Figure 46: A female healer attends an inauguration ceremony

underlies the healing can be amplified to some extent through Jung's concept of *synchronicity*. Jung coined the term synchronicity to demonstrate that psyche and matter exist as one reality, where matter, at times, responds as spirit, and spirit manifests in matter.

Synchronicity

The red threads throughout this book link the phenomena of union of opposites, acausal orderedness, absolute knowledge in the collective unconscious, natural numbers, and the unity of matter and psyche. These potentially are woven into a discernable whole in Jung's concept of synchronicity. Von Franz (1992, p. 40) explained that with the creation of the concept of synchronicity, "Jung laid a foundation which may lead us to see the complementary realms of psyche and matter." Von Franz continues that "synchronistic events thus seem to point towards a *unitary aspect of existence* which transcends our conscious grasp and which Jung called the *unus mundus*."

A precise definition of synchronicity, according to von Franz (1992) requires the coincidence of two psychic states: the causal event perceived by our senses in the outer world and the impression that this outer event is "interrupted by an archetypally conditioned constellation" (p. 209). Jung (1952c) cautioned that synchronistic events are not "caused" by any archetype, rather through a synchronistic happening, the nascent meaning of the archetype emerges (para. 965).

In essence, through the *ukuthwasa* experience, the archetype of the Self is activated. Evidence of this is apparent in an increase in synchronistic happenings on the outer aspect, which often symbolize a deeper connection with the collective unconscious. Von Franz (1980b) explained that when an archetype is activated it has a direct impact on the conscious situation (p. 54). Thus the archetype could be defined as a structure which "conditions certain psychological probabilities . . . which underlies a synchronistic event . . . [which is] not predictable precisely because it is always a creative act in time" (1980b, p. 54).

Jung cautioned that we only speak of the effect of archetypal phenomenon when two conditions are present and related: image and emotion. He noted that when the archetypal image "is charged with numinosity . . . with psychic energy . . . it becomes dynamic and will produce consequences" (1961b, para. 589). In archetypal situations such as death, illness, and the *ukuthwasa* phenomenon, the threshold of consciousness is lowered due to heightened emotions, and the unconscious and its contents gain an upper hand. This is often the precondition for synchronistic events. Jung (1952c) observed that "the medicine man has the capacity which cannot be explained scientifically. He is capable of raising himself to an extreme level of emotion through conscious act of will, creating the conditions necessary for synchronistic events" (para. 859).

In synchronistic phenomena, which characterize much of the African healing realm, there is a merging of time, space, image, and object wherein something of the transcendental unity becomes visible. This phenomenon is the essential underlying factor in the success of the healing rituals. Synchronistic experiences demand of us the realization that matter trans- gresses into the realm of spirit and spirit into the realm of matter. Through the merging of the physical and the nonphysical, the manifestation of spirit in matter and matter in spirit, held in the retort of the healer-ancestor unity, healing can manifest.

Von Franz (1999) described this phenomenon within the psycho- therapeutic vessel and stated that "an archetypal experience is the only healing factor in therapy . . . if it does not happen, you cannot do much" (p. 9). Jung (1961b) observed the effect of the activation of the archetypal energies when he stated that "the archetype is a piece of life, an image connected to the living individual by a bridge of emotion" (para. 589).

Jung (1954a) differentiated between two poles in the sphere of the totality of the psyche (para. 343). He called the one pole the ultraviolet end of the scale with the opposite pole being the infrared end. On the ultraviolet end, Jung investigated the archetypes in the psychological forms or manifestations: how archetypes appear in dreams and in unconscious images; in other words, the realm of mind and spirit. On the infrared end, Jung was referring to the archetypal image as located in the material aspect of the psyche, the realm of emotions and impulses to act; the realm of body and matter. Both the infrared and ultraviolet poles affect and influence each other. At the ultraviolet pole, certain material phenomena occur: These are the so-called parapsychological phenomena. On the infrared pole, some- thing psychic can simultaneously express itself materially.

The distinction is academic, as the poles are points in the sphere of the totality of the psyche. Matter sometimes shows up at the ultraviolet pole and vice versa. What we designate as matter or energy in the external world are both archetypal images. What I am concerned with here is how these actualize in an experience in consciousness. The interaction between matter and spirit is an occurrence that has existed in the mythology and philosophies of antiquity and is certainly alive and well in the epistemology of the healers. More recently, this is now emerging as a concept in modern physics and quantum mechanics. David Bohm (1980), the physicist, postulated the indivisibility of all material processes. Essentially he said that "all observable matter in the universe is the explicate order of an underlying enfolded implicate order," in other words, an undifferentiated wholeness (p. 197). He further postulated that matter in general, and consciousness in particular, may have this explicate/manifest order in common, a unity of all existence, an infinite reservoir of energy that lies behind our consciousness. Modern scientific developments seem to indicate a tendency in physical theory to recognize that something psychic and material could be two aspects of the same foundation.[19]

In the postulations about the paradoxes of the uncertainty principle, the observer effect is the label given to the fact that it is impossible to carry out an observation of something independent of the influence of the observer. Von Franz (1986) cites Pauli who defined physical knowledge as the meeting of inner psychological images and outer facts (p. 20).

Synchronistic and empirically inexplicable events occur when one enters the realm of African healing, enough to convince most of us that these phenomena do exist, even though as yet we have no rational explanation for them. Nonetheless, that these occur autonomously seems plausible. It is not possible to always explain or reduce these occurrences to projections of complexes. Rather, it appears that the authenticity of these experiences need to be held as autonomous phenomena independent of, but also related to, our subjective worlds.

For the African healer, most events have some meaning. Illnesses, accidents, and good fortune are not considered arbitrary acts of chance, but are understood as meaningful coincidences. This understanding echoes Jung's (1952c) concept of synchronicity "the simultaneous occurrence of two meaningful, but not causally connected events" (para. 849). The meaningful connection between the two states is usually only apparent after the passage of time. That is, in hindsight, it becomes clear that there was a connection between seemingly arbitrary events (for an example, see chapter 9 and the description of the snake at my door). This reflects the idea that there is a kind of knowledge or consciousness in the archetypal realm, not yet known to ego consciousness until an image or an event breaks through.

The observation of synchronistic phenomena led Jung to postulate the link between psyche and matter. Jung noted that the psyche could be regarded as a quality of matter and matter as a concrete aspect of the psyche. Nature contains everything: therefore, all unknown things, including matter. For Jung (1977):

> The empirical world is in a sense appearance, that is to say it is related to another order of things below it or behind it. Where "here" and "there" do not exist; where there is no extension in space, which means space does not exist, and no extension in time, which means time does not exist. . . . We must face the fact that something of our psychic existence is outside space and time, that is, beyond changeability. (p. 378)

Here, too, the phenomenon of natural numbers, as noted with respect to the sacrificial rituals, is relevant. Von Franz (1974) noted that "all numbers are simply qualitatively differentiated manifestations of the primal one . . . a mathematical symbol of the *unus mundus*" (p. 66). Von Franz (1992) later elaborated that "numbers . . . represent the actual matrix of the archetype. . . . [and] point to a background of reality in which psyche and matter are no longer distinguishable" (p. 216). This background reality is what Jung (1975) called "a world-system whose space-time categories are relatively or absolutely abolished" (p. 399). Jung continued, noting that number may be the key to the mystery of the *unus mundus* in that "it is quantity as well as meaning."

My thesis here is to suggest that the progressive unfolding of the stages of the *ukuthwasa* initiation essentially reflects an archetypal image of a creative process that strives to establish an orientation toward wholeness in the initiate. As von Franz (1992) explained:

> When any archetype constellates, it first manifests as *one* archetypal image . . . When it moves toward the threshold of consciousness it generally appears doubled. . . . Three groups . . .

symbolize that that very archetype is possessing the ego. . . . When the same content appears in its four-phase it has reached its best possibility for being realized in our consciousness. (pp. 283–284)

During the *ukuthwasa* initiation, as reflected in each stage, there is a cessation of focus on outer activities and everything is put into the retort, so to say, of the ritual. It is then, as noted by von Franz (1997b) that "the experience of the self is expressed as one's innermost soul, which is touched by the dynamic aspect of the God-image, through meditative contemplation and introversion, the unconscious . . . begins to flow" (p. 48). Thus the *ukuthwasa* state is a temporary, artificial state of complete introversion with the required concentration of libido on the inner life. This process, if followed carefully, potentially births a new symbol of the Self.

An additional mystery is the question of what *is* healing, which undoubtedly arises when one engages with this material. In relation to synchronicity, healing can be understood as *"acts of creation in time"* (Jung, 1934a, para. 965). Von Franz (1992) distinguished between healing that is causal, that is, a result of an interaction between psyche and matter, and healing with respect to synchronicity. She states that "only processes involved in 'miraculous' cures, which are unpredictable, can be understood as synchronistic incidents" (p. 249). The healing in the realm of the African healer seems to embody the latter. The *ukuthwasa* phenomenon places the healer at the point of contact where psyche and matter meet, and healing is an observable outcome of this contact. Von Franz (1974) explained further:

The mysterious point of contact between the two systems appears to be the center or sort of pivot where psyche and matter meet. When an individual enters into relation with the forces of the pivot, he finds himself close to the sphere of "miracles." . . . When such a constellation exists and eternity breaks though momentarily into our temporal system, the primal unity actively manifests itself and . . . unites . . . into one. . . . This is how the *unus mundus* becomes revealed in the phenomenon of synchronicity. (p. 263)

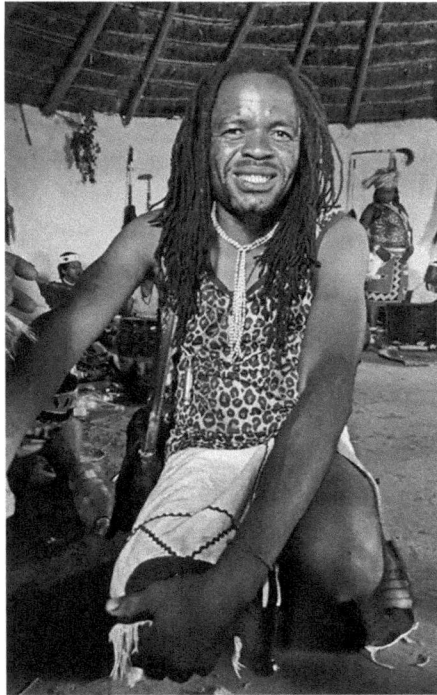

Figure 47: A male healer rests in the initiation hut after an inauguration ceremony

The Stages of the *Coniunctio*

It gradually dawned on me that the potential outcome of the initiation experience is the facilitation of opposites coming together and reflecting the mystery of the *coniunctio.*[20] I contemplated the impact of the initiation with respect to becoming conscious of the larger inner presence while giving the utmost care to the unconscious and to nature. As expressed by Jung (1955–56), the reconciliation of the tension of opposites allows for the emergence of the harmonious "third" and can be said to be part of a new inner God-image (para. 206). And further, as Jung (1975) explained, "a restitution of the original oneness of the unconscious on the level of consciousness" (p. 135). In this light, Edinger (quoted in Jaffe, 1991) elaborated that the goal of individuation is "the *coniunctio.* The time has come for the psychic opposites, heaven and earth, male and female, spirit and nature, good and evil, which have long been torn asunder in the Western psyche, to be reconciled" (p. 49).

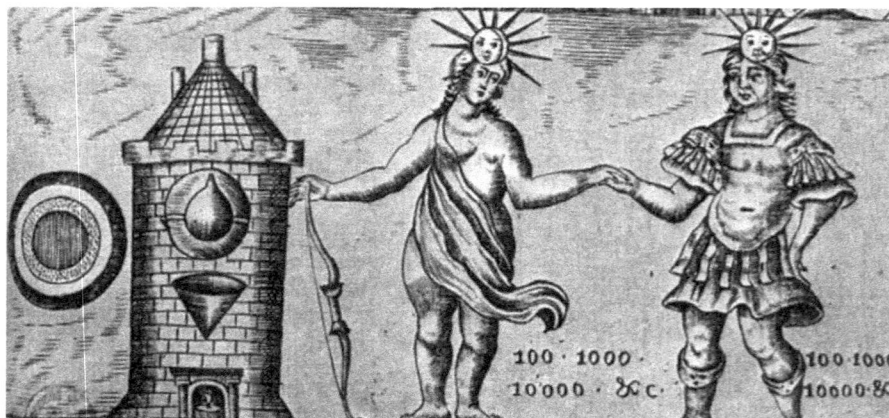

Figure 48: The *coniunctio* of opposites symbolized by the male and female pair.
Mutus Liber, pl. 10

The symbol of the *coniunctio* plays a central part in the alchemical opus as Jung (1946b) noted: "The idea of the *coniunctio* . . . became the symbol of the *unio mystica* . . . the archetype of the union of opposites—the change from a *disiunctio* into a *coniunctio*" (para. 354).

Building further on the amplification of the Zulu initiation with respect to individuation and the alchemical process, the stages of the initiation embody the stages of the *coniunctio* identified by the alchemist Dorn (Gerhard Dorneus, 1530/34 - ca.1584). As Jung (1955–56) outlined, these stages of the *coniunctio* consist first of the *unio mentalis*, followed by the uniting of the *unio mentalis* with the body—the *unio corporalis*—and culminating in the *unus mundus*. The stages of the *ukuthwasa* initiation also can be understood to embody this threefold *coniunctio*, as each stage carries within it a level of transformation for the initiate.

As we have seen, the individual whose fate it is to become a healer is usually identified through an initiatory illness and begins in a state of darkness akin to the alchemical *nigredo*. The function of the *nigredo* has a double meaning embedded in such experiences, as highlighted by Jung, which includes the significance of such a period of darkness with respect to transformation. Thus the *nigredo* is at the same time something divine wherein the embryo of the healer incubates.

Edinger (1995) explained that such an event in one's life is "a calling from out of the darkness and the abyss, and if the ego attends to that call it will be given a connection with the morning star" (p. 209). In other words, the recognition and engagement with the *nigredo* is the precondition toward transformation and individuation. Edinger (1995) goes on to explain that the double meaning of the *nigredo* is

> praising God from the depths because one has been given the capacity to look into the deep things of God. So we have a double meaning, then, of the depths: on the one side it means to fall into the fog and the darkness and to be inundated by the waters; and at the same time it means to be initiated into the deep things of God. Psychologically, this means that an encounter with the unconscious brings first darkness, disorientation and distress; but if one persists in scrutinizing the experience, its consequence is to enlarge the personality and bring one closer to wholeness. (pp. 209–210)

This beginning of the transformation on an individual level is often announced by the *nigredo*, and in the African healing realm this state initiates the phenomenon of the calling. Individually, for Ntombi, as we have seen, this meant the loss of meaning in her artificially imposed religious doctrine, and the beginning of her transformation toward individuation. Alchemically, the *nigredo* state is the precursor to the emergence of the first *coniunctio*.

The *Unio Mentalis*

The darkening or *nigredo* stage of the *ukuthwasa* initiation is the pre-condition that heralds the whitening, akin to the alchemical *albedo*. Here the focus is on the union of the soul of the initiate with the spirit of the ancestors. This stage is referred to as the spiritualization stage. The body is dealt with aesthetically with severe restrictions of food, drink, clothing, and bodily needs, as well as a period of celibacy. The initiate experiences this stage as a kind of nonbeing, a loss of all previous states of being, a return to a state from which something is reborn. The healers explain that at this time all outer distractions are minimized so that the initiate can focus on the relationship to the ancestors without contaminations. Jung (1955–56) described this stage as follows:

The mind (*mens*) must be separated from the body—which is equivalent to "voluntary death"—for only separated things can unite. . . . The aim of this separation was to free the mind from the influence of "bodily appetites and the heart's affections," and to establish a spiritual position which is subordinate to the turbulent sphere of the body. (para. 671)

During this stage, which begins with withdrawal, restraint, restrictions, and isolation, Ntombi was required to await a visitation from the ancestral spirits with whom she engages in her mind. Thus this first stage is an imaginary one. Von Franz (1974), discussing Dorn's trinity of the *coniunctio*, explained that this begins with

a kind of alchemistic meditation in which the instinctual aspect of the body was first to be subdued, by separating soul and spirit from it. Then soul and spirit were to be fused into a *unio mentalis* in order to be reunited subsequently with the purified body. (p. 261)

This is the first *coniunctio*, the *unio mentalis* (mental union) described by Dorn, and which Jung (1955–56) explained as referring "to the union of the soul and the spirit which are separated from the body" (para. 673). Here, the soul unites with spirit in an interior oneness. This involves the withdrawal of projections from the bodily sphere and from all environmental conditions relating to the body.

At this time, by observing the strict restrictions of the whitening stage, Ntombi became aware or conscious of the ancestral voices within, confronting parts of her personality that had been acquired or contaminated by shadow aspects. Here, she confronted her beliefs about herself and her awareness of her intention in participating in the initiation. This beginning stage opens the communication with the ancestors, ensuring the efficacy of the initiate-ancestor relationship. As Jung (1955–56) noted, "the *unio mentalis* then in psychological . . . language means knowledge of oneself . . . the self as a substance incommensurable with the ego, hidden in the body, and identical with the image of God" (para. 711).

Dorn taught that alchemically, once the objective standpoint of the *unio mentalis* has been achieved, the liberated spirit/soul *coniunctio* must be united with the matter once again. This entails the reconnection with the body, the *unio corporalis*, a "coming down to earth" and a *coagulatio.*

The *Unio Corporalis*

The reddening of the *ukuthwasa* initiation, as noted previously, is referred to as the full-blooded stage, akin to the alchemical *rubedo*. This stage includes a return of the libido, the end of the celibacy period, the mixing of the blood with the *muthi*. In the second stage of the *coniunctio,* the *unio mentalis* is reunited with the body. This signals a return of the spirit/soul union to the body and an embodiment of the psyche and matter. As Jung (1955–56) outlined:

> The reuniting of the *unio mentalis* with the body, is particularly important, as only here can the complete conjunction be attained—union with the *unus mundus*. The reuniting of the spiritual position with the body obviously means that the insights gained should be made real. (para. 679)

This stage is one of difficulty and conflict resulting in a synthesis of conscious and unconscious. Edinger (1995) reflecting on this stage, notes that it "involves bringing the consciousness of wholeness, which in the first stage is a kind of abstract realization, into a full-blooded reality so that one lives it out fully in everyday life" (p. 296). This mirrors the stages of the initiation from the whitening, through the reddening to the many-colored stage symbolized by the changes in the outer regalia of the initiate.

At this stage, the blood of the animal is significant and is used in some of the initiatory regalia. Jung (1955–56) explained that in alchemy blood symbolizes the "powerful medicine for uniting the *unio mentalis* with the body" (para. 690). The blood is one essential facet of the *unio corporalis*—that which brings the *unio mentalis* and the body back together. Blood is the vital life essence, the divine fluid, symbolic of the covenant and cementing the connection between God and man. The symbolism of blood and the relationship to spirit is found across a number of religions as well as myths and legends. We can think of Abel's blood that calls out from the earth after he is slain by Cain. In the myth of Odysseus where the blood of the sacrificed sheep poured on the ground attracts the spirits of the dead. In alchemical terms, blood is synonymous with the "*aqua permanens* and spirit" and Dorn spoke of blood as the "redeeming substance" (Jung, 1955–56, para. 401).

Psychologically, the blood sacrifice symbolizes how the unconscious is brought into contact with consciousness. The assimilation of the potency of the animal through eating its flesh and blood and wearing its skin is a convergence of the natural and supernatural, the healer and ancestor, personal and transpersonal. The spirit embodied in the flesh must be treated in this way in order to ensure renewal. For the healer, this stage is accompanied by the ability to affect the healing on a physical level as well as a spiritual level. For Ntombi this stage represented her resolution of her inner conflict, resulting in her full embodiment of her cultural heritage and her more authentic self-image.

The *Unus Mundus* or *Unio Mystica*

Dorn identified the final stage of the *coniunctio* as the united spirit-soul-body with the world, the *unus mundus*. Here, Dorn referred to the uniting with the one world of the beginning of creation. This stage is only possible after reuniting spirit/soul and body/matter in stage two. As Jung (1955–56) expanded, the self enters three-dimensional reality when the ego touches the potential world, the *unus mundus*. To contemplate the third *coniunctio* is potentially to tread on uncharted and treacherous territory. Jung (1955–56) cautioned that "even Dorn did not venture to assert that he or any other adept had perfected the third stage in his lifetime" (para. 666). To approach the third coniunctio here, is to hint at the potential embedded in the symbolism of the *unus mundus* and not to assert any realizable goal. Edinger (1995) elaborated:

> At this level, time and eternity are united and synchronicity prevails . . . this is a borderline state that one can only glimpse from afar . . . the assumption is that final and total transition to unity is consummated only at death. (p. 281)

And further:

> The third phase—the creation or realization of the *unus mundus*—
> is a transcendent symbolic condition that defies any com-
> prehensive or adequate description. It refers to a superlative
> experience of unity in which subject and object, inner and outer,
> are transcended in the experience of a unitary reality really
> beyond our grasp. (p. 296)

As mentioned previously, the noticeable feature of the African healing system is the phenomenon of synchronicity, which as Jung taught, is a feature of the state of *unus mundus*, the unity of spirit and matter. Jung (1955–56) observed:

> If a union is to take place between opposites like spirit and matter,
> conscious and unconscious, bright and dark . . . it will happen in a
> third thing, which represents not a compromise but something
> new . . . by a transcendental entity that could be described only
> in paradoxes. (para. 765)

As we have reflected, synchronicity is one possible phenomenon that underlies the healing effect in this cosmology, that of the healer's affinity with both spirit and matter and the influence of one on the other in a reciprocal union. In extrapolating from the work of the alchemists in general and the work of Dorn in particular, Jung demonstrated that the third level of the *coniunctio* is one that has universal applicability. Jung (1955–56) stated, "the thought that Dorn expresses by the third degree of conjunction . . . is the relation or identity of the personal with the suprapersonal atman, and of the individual Tao with the universal Tao" (para. 762).

Jung further acknowledged, as is often the case with the African healing realm, that to the Western mind this concept appears to be too "mystical." However, he reiterated that such a perception is indicative of a lack of experience on the part of the Westerner. He states that "it is chiefly our ignorance of the psyche if these experiences appear 'mystic'" (1955–56, para. 762).

Once again, the phenomenon of psyche and matter and spirit in nature emerges through the third *coniunctio* and the *unus mundus*. Jung (1955–56) explained:

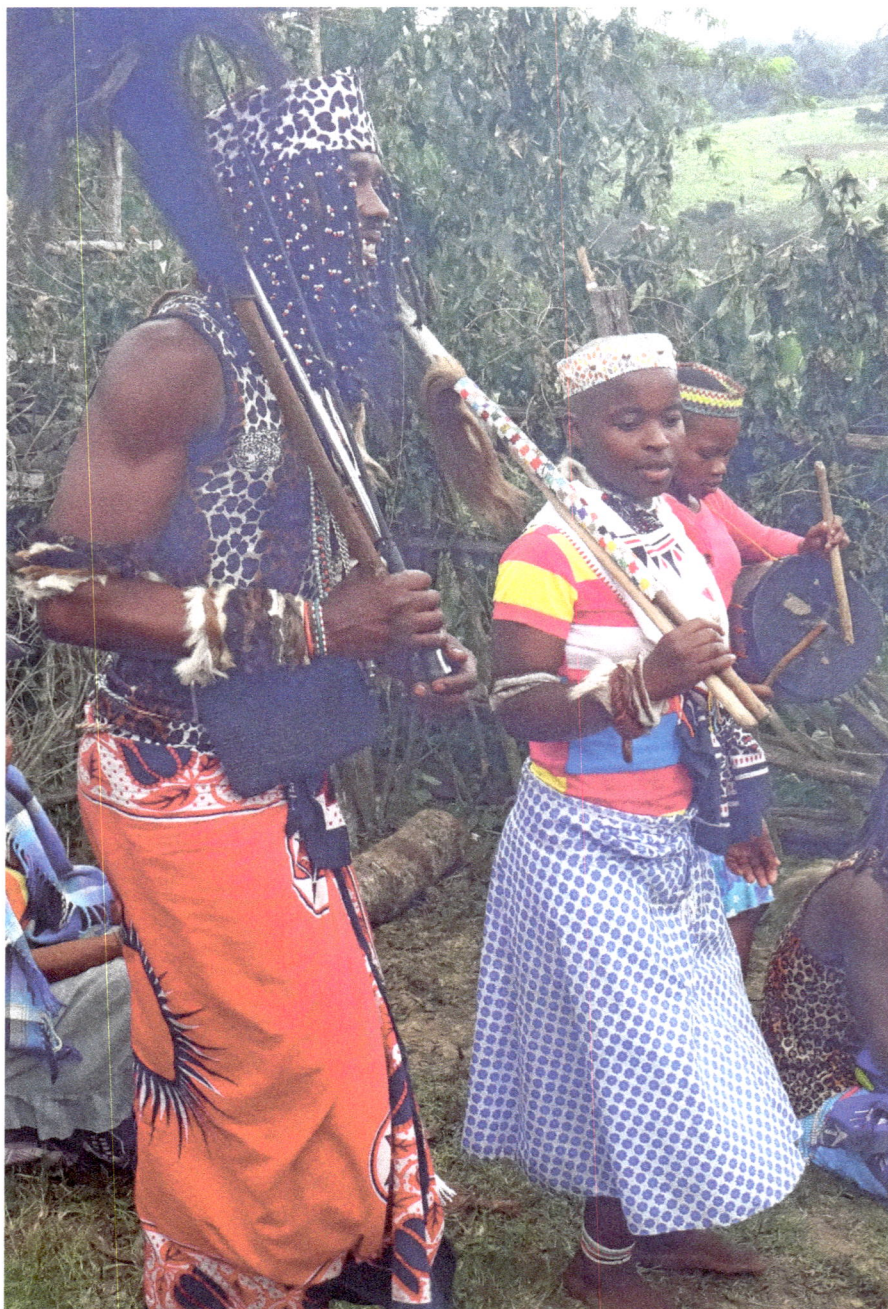

Figure 49. Senior male healer and his *thwasa*, now healer, dance at the end of her graduation ceremony

Undoubtedly the idea of the *unus mundus* is founded on the assumption that the multiplicity of the empirical world rests on an underlying unity. . . . That even the psychic world, which is so extraordinarily different from the physical world, does not have its roots outside the one cosmos is evident from the undeniable fact that causal connections exist between the psyche and the body which point to their underlying unitary nature. (para. 767)

This encapsulates the phenomenon of the African healer's abilities and the culmination of Ntombi's healing. Through a carefully nurtured relationship between the healer and the ancestors, the preservation of the relationship between the individual and the transcendental, a transformation on the physical as well as on the spiritual plane is possible. The healers are very clear about this relationship, and symptoms of illness or dis-ease are symbolic of disruptions in this balance. Here, the final stage of transformation of the third *coniunctio* reflects the emergence of the fully evolved healer.

Concluding Reflections

In essence, what I have hoped to convey in this work is the idea of the evolution of consciousness in the individual through the initiation, culminating in a connection to an inner numinous God-image. As such, in my view, this phenomenon can be understood psychologically as an image of the individuation process and development in consciousness, as for the African healer this ritual initiates and fulfils the personal transformation. This transformation seems to provide a connection between outer and inner life. The numinous archetypal images that manifest in the inner visions and dream world of the initiate are distilled, coagulated, and digested and emerge in a lived experience.

Here, we potentially meet the ultimate challenge faced in analysis: that of how to bridge the relationship between the archetypal and the personal, which then has a consequence for the individual. Or how to encourage a living relationship between the inner and outer realms of the individual that potentially results in a greater capacity for differentiation, for relatedness, and for consciousness. Unless this makes a difference in life, it remains but an elusive abstraction. For the African healer, to be touched by the archetype is essentially to see and be seen by the Godhead, the unconscious, and thus to gain validity.

In my attempt to bridge the divide between my Western-based analytical training and knowledge gained from my experiences within the African healing realm, such a relationship between symptoms of dis-ease and the transpersonal world became more and more apparent.

An example of this occurred in a particularly difficult analytical session with Ntombi. Her inner conflict had resulted in another episode of depression and I felt a sense of despair. She had expressed repeated suicidal ideations and her helplessness, and mine in assisting her, was immense. In this session, I had a vision. She was sitting on the chair in front of me, and to her left, high above her head, was a bright circular light. The light shattered into many splinters and fell down under the earth. I knew that I would need to collect the splinters if there was to be any hope for Ntombi. I asked her to sit quietly and not to speak. I felt myself descend into the darkness, searching for the splinters of light. Each time I found one, I returned to her and asked her to swallow it. This went on many times repeatedly until there seemed to be no more splinters left in the underworld. It felt like many months had passed, but in reality, only one hour of real time had elapsed. I did not tell her of my experience immediately, as I felt I needed time to process the experience. The following day, Ntombi called me to say she had had a dream in which, as she related it to me, was the exact experience of my vision. Her healing progressed rapidly thereafter; she was able to engage more fully in her process in both realms: that of the analytical temenos and the initiatory realm.

In this experience, the autonomy and the mystery of the psyche seemed most palpable. I was aware that I had not engaged in this process through an act of will, but rather I was, unwittingly, a conduit for something to emerge that could be harnessed and made available to Ntombi for her own healing. It required the reflected response from her unconscious in the form of her dream for the cycle to be complete. Von Franz (1997b) observes "when an archetype is intensely constellated in the unconscious, outer events happen" (p. 56).

Jung (1954a) cited Dorn's observation of the "star-like sparks" that appear during the alchemical operations, which symbolize the light of God (a similar phenomenon is found in both the Jewish Kabbalistic creation myth as well as the Gnostic myth of reintegrating light sparks). Jung explained that the concept of the divine sparks "have clear psychological meaning for Dorn. This light is the *lumen naturae*, which illuminates consciousness, and the *scintellae* are germinal luminosities shining forth from the darkness of the unconscious" (para. 389).

In the realm of African healing, we meet, I believe the mysterious knowledge in nature, the *lumen naturae* that the alchemists spoke of, and which we psychologically experience as the inner knowledge of the unconscious. Here, in this realm, the luminous knowledge of the unconscious is a lived experience that hints at the ineffable mystery of the totality. Jung (1942) observed that "Nature is not matter only, she is also spirit . . . The *lumen naturae* is the natural spirit whose strange and significant workings we can observe in the manifestations of the unconscious . . . an autonomous psychic system." (para. 229)

Psychologically, this seems to suggest a model for the ego in relationship to the unconscious: to become conscious of, not ego desires and thoughts, but the great inner wisdom of the *lumen naturae*, the *anima mundi*, a numinous impersonal layer of the psyche, related to the personal, but not identical to it. To quote Edinger (1984):

> As it gradually dawns on people one by one that the transformation of God is not just an interesting idea, but is a living reality, it may begin to function as a new myth. Whoever recognizes this myth as his own personal reality will put his life in the service of this process. Such an individual offers himself as a vessel for the incarnation of the deity and thereby promotes the ongoing transformation of God by giving Him human manifestation. Such an individual will experience his life as meaningful. (p. 113)

The journey into the world of the African healer became, for me, the discovery that what appears irrational is also rational, both concrete and abstract, symbolic and actual and hints at the lawfulness of the autonomous psyche. The relatedness to these people and their deeply spiritual way of life offers us a unique gift of touching and being touched by the archetypal material, and not only the symbolic language embedded in these experiences, but also how these precious gifts can be brought back into consciousness or actuality.

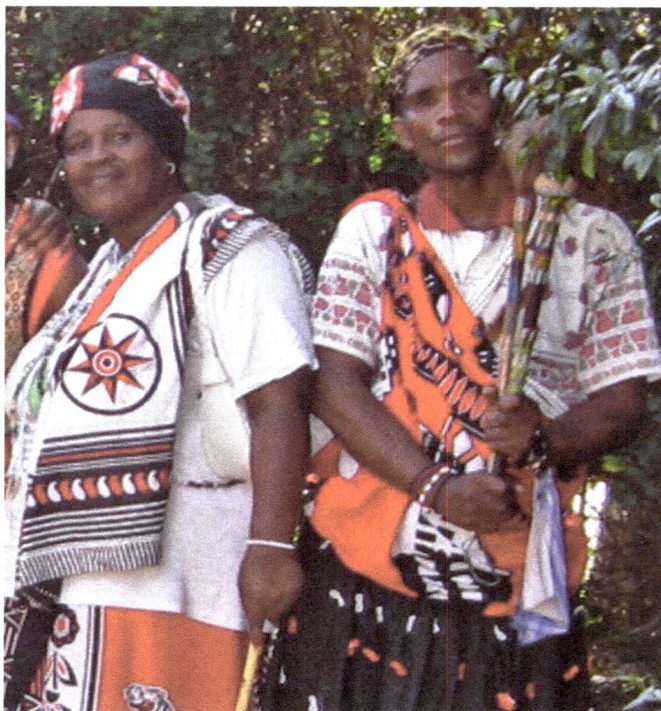

Figure 50: A male and female *sangoma* couple

In this realm, the aspect of our natures that seems to have been left behind in the pursuit of rational consciousness is alive and well: That of the instinctual aspect of life symbolized by the animal, where the gods were once animals, animals were once people, and people become animals. Jung (2008) noted that the oldest psychic representations of our instincts are the animal gods. Jung elaborated that the "animal is a pious, law abiding being who fulfills the will of god in the most perfect way . . . It seems to have direct access to some power which it honors with a divine devotion." (p.37)

It is no longer natural for us to understand the meaning behind the animal symbol. Von Franz (1997a) reminds us that "we have to descend quite far down into ourselves . . . in order to be able to understand the animal . . . and when we do we discover that they reflect the very most primal of our unconscious psyche." (p. 112)

My experience of witnessing the healer's fidelity to spirit, humility in the face of the autonomous psyche, and their acceptance of nature brought home me to the realization of the imperative to hold and traverse these realms, to accept how the darkness potentially transforms, and that it is this transformation that can lead to healing. I became aware of my doubts, which often took the form of recurring questions: Do I know how to recognize the potential meaning in suffering? Am I aware of how essential it is to be related to something greater, where the very way of life is to be connected to a personal myth, which is related to a universal myth? Am I capable of navigating the wounding in others in the analytical vessel? How do I hold the experience that it is this very wounding that often becomes the path to healing? How do we nurture this mysterious process of the reality of the inner wisdom of the unconscious psyche? If I am not conscious of these aspects, how can I dare to witness the suffering, with the resultant potential transformation, of my patients?

With these questions in mind and through the work with Ntombi, I realized the importance, not only of theoretical knowledge but also, of being personally involved in my own inner work and experiences. During this time of writing, the following dream image appeared as compensation to my recurring doubts and seemed to reflect Ntombi's journey: A voice says: "Read page p. 753 of Jung's visions." I woke and immediately went to get the book. This paragraph stood out for me:

> You may have an ego will . . . you are attracted by something outside . . . [but] it will be contradicted by the archetypal law of the collective unconscious that life must evolve in a certain way. . . . The archetypal law often seems to us like defeat, a standstill. Most people get terribly impatient and even despair because nothing happens, they get nowhere, they are all the time hindered, they don't understand that this is just as it must be and actually their only chance to get there. . . . As long as the non-ego seems to be in opposition to the ego, you feel it naturally as an opposite, but you will understand after a while that that the collective unconscious is like a wide sea, and the ego is like a little boat drifting upon it. (In C.G. Jung, 1997b, p. 753)

Through honoring the work of transformation in the individual, this in turn potentially could have a reciprocal effect on collective consciousness. Jung (1957b) notes "if the individual is not truly regenerated in spirit, society cannot be either" (para. 536). Here Jung is commenting on the need for the healing of the split so visible in the collective consciousness of the day. We still see evidence of this split on a daily basis: the increase in fundamentalist attitudes, radical terrorist brutality, intolerance and fear of "otherness," and the breakdown of systems—both economic and religious—reflected in nature, and in the climatic shifts that are a reality today. It is only by recognizing that the outer divisions are reflective of an inner division that salvation may be possible. Jung (1957b) wrote, "anyone who has insight into his own actions, and thus has found access to the unconscious . . . exercises an influence on his environment" (para. 583). Von Franz (1980a) extrapolated:

> In the final analysis it is consciousness that makes the conflict between the inner and the outer by projecting the one as materially real and the other as psychically real, because we do not really know the difference between material reality and the psyche. We are confronted with something unknown which appears sometimes as matter and sometimes as psyche. It is a life mystery, which seems to manifest both psychologically and materially. If we describe it from the outside . . . it appears as matter, and if we approach it from within it appears as what we like to call the unconscious. (p. 147)

For the African healer, the realm of this mystery carries an additional dimension in that it has a manifest reality deeply rooted in a living experience. Jung (1946c) stressed that "it . . . behooves us . . . to go to school once more with the medical philosophers [and the indigenous healers] of a distant past, when body and soul had not yet been wrenched asunder into different faculties" (para. 190). And further, Jung (1954b) recommends that we

> turn back to those periods in human history when symbol formation still went on unimpeded, that is, when there was still no epistemological criticism of the formation of images, and when, in consequence, facts that in themselves were unknown could be expressed in definite visual form. (para. 353)

I am grateful to have witnessed these healing rituals and to have been offered a glimpse of this ineffable mystery. I am left with the inevitable conclusion that what is being embodied in the African healer's initiation is an image of that interrelationship between spirit and matter that we talk about. This is, for me, a *coniunctio* in the most profound. To deal with the *coniunctio* in human words is a disconcerting task, since you are forced to express and formulate a process taking place beyond the sphere of discriminating consciousness.

Approaching this mysterious and somewhat incomprehensible phenomenon, I am reminded of Jung's (1975) words when he wrote, in relation to the *coniunctio* mystery: "I cannot confess to have solved the riddle of the *coniunctio* mystery. On the contrary I am darkly aware of things lurking in the background of the problem—things too big for our horizons" (p. 393). However Jung (1955-56) is encouraging when he says:

> One should not be put off by the physical impossibilities of the *coniunctio*, . . . for [it] is a symbol in regard to which the allurements of rationalism are entirely out of place. . . . If symbols mean anything at all, they are tendencies which pursue a definite but not yet recognizable goal and consequently can express themselves only in analogies. (para. 667)

In essence, as summarized by von Franz (1980a):

> the *coniunctio* . . . ends with an incarnation of the Divinity, it is God coming down into the human being. That is what Jung formulated in saying that what is seen from the human angle as being the process of individuation, as seen from the angle of the image of God is a process of incarnation. (p. 272)

Reflecting on Ntombi and her fear as her overriding symptom, I recalled Jung's words: "where the fear, there is your task" (1975, p. 306). It was this fear that ultimately became the vessel for the transformation needed with respect to Ntombi's inner conflict. The fear led to its antinomy, in that Ntombi recognized the opposite face of her fear, that of the numinous inner face of the God-image. As von Franz (1997a) observed: "If we suffer the problem of opposites to the utmost and accept it into ourselves, we can sometimes become a place in which opposites can spontaneously come together." Jung (1944) concluded, "without the experience of opposites there is no experience of wholeness and hence no inner approach to the sacred figures" (para. 24).

To give a full description of the wealth of the symbols embedded in the initiatory process or in the alchemical opus is beyond the scope of this work. My intention was to moisten the imagination while lending validity and honor to the courage of Ntombi during what could be called her *peregrinatio*, her pilgrimage back to her heritage. Ultimately, the desired outcome of the work, be it the alchemical opus, the African healing initiation, or the work in analysis, is that of striving for wholeness, a balance of opposites, and a greater sense of Self. As Jung (1946b) reminds us: "Is there anything more fundamental than the realization, 'This is what I am'? . . . No longer the earlier ego with its make-believes and artificial contrivances, but another, 'objective' ego . . . better called the 'self.'" (para. 400).

Ntombi went on to complete her initiation into the realms of the Zulu healer as well as her medical training within the biomedical system. Her aim was to somehow bridge the divide between these two modalities and to contribute in some small way to the harmony beyond the tension of opposites.

Appendix
A Brief Account of the
South African Demographic

The latest census puts the total population of South Africa at approximately 59,000,000, with an average life expectancy of almost 60 years. Christianity is the dominant religion, followed by Islam. Currently, the black people make up about 80 percent of the population and are representative of four major ethnic groups: Nguni, Sotho, Shangaan-Tsonga, and Venda. The Nguni comprise two-thirds of the black population and are subdivided into four groups: Zulu, Xhosa, Swazi, and Ndebele. What is important to note is that although there are broad similarities, these different tribes are disparate and individual, with their own languages, cultural belief systems, and practices. People from one tribe do not necessarily speak or understand the language from another tribe. Such is the complexity and multicultural context of Africa and South Africa.

The white people constitute a little over 9 percent of the population and include decedents from Portuguese, Dutch, French, German, and British colonists, as well as more recent immigrants. The colored people make up another 9 percent of the population and are the mixed-race people, historically descended from the early white settlers, indigenous peoples, and slaves. In addition, there is a small Indian population of about 2.5 percent. South Africa has 11 official languages, which include English and the local Afrikaans, derived from Dutch and German, as well as nine indigenous languages.

The Original People

The genetic heritage of *Homo sapiens* can be traced to the early hominids that roamed Africa. The paleontological importance of Africa is well-established, with southern Africa referred to as "the cradle of humankind." The original people were the Bushmen, who seem to have been the earliest people to migrate south from central Africa to the tip of the African continent. Vestiges of the cultural and spiritual practices of the Bushmen are found in the African healing systems. Skilled hunter-gatherers and nomads, the Bushmen had great respect for the land, and their lifestyle had a low environmental impact, allowing them to sustain their way of life without leaving much archaeological evidence. Other than the well-known rock paintings, etchings, and petroglyphs, the Bushmen left little trace of their early culture.

Carbon dating of relics that were found, place Bushmen activity as early as 80,000–100,000 years ago. A small number of Bushmen still live in South Africa and southern Africa, making them the oldest continuously existing culture in the world, closely followed by the Aboriginal Australians.

Different migratory routes resulted in the Bushmen developing into two distinct groups: the pastoral Bushmen, known as the KhoiKhoi, and the hunter-gathers, known as the San. The KhoiKhoi migrated to the coastal areas, and the San remained in the interior. Today there are small groups of Bushmen in Namibia and the Kalahari. Intermarriage between the two tribes resulted in today's remaining tribe, known as the KhoiSan. Sadly, due to a combination of intermarriage and persecution by black tribes and white European settlers, the Bushmen are no longer a pure race, and few recall the ancient healing practices of their ancestors.

Black Migration

Archaeological data suggests that almost 2,500 years ago, the black tribes migrated to southern Africa from the Great Lakes regions. The Great Lakes are a series of lakes in and around the Great Rift Valley and include Lake Victoria, the second-largest freshwater lake in the world and the source of the Nile and Lake Tanganyika, the second-deepest lake in the world. The Great Lakes region encompasses Burundi, Rwanda, the Democratic Republic of Congo, Uganda, Kenya, and Tanzania.

The black people started to make their way south and east around 1,000 B.C. and reached the east coast of South Africa in about 500 A.D. They were an advanced Iron Age culture, practicing agriculture, including animal husbandry and farming, and they lived in settled villages. The migratory groups formed the ancestors to today's Nguni tribes.

Colonization and the Arrival of the White Man

The Portuguese were the first Europeans to arrive on the east coast of Africa in 1488, and they settled in Mozambique, establishing trade routes with India and China. They enjoyed sole proprietorship until the 16th century and the arrival of the English and the Dutch. The sea routes around the southern tip of Africa became more popular and the Cape became a regular stopover point. Cape Point, known as the Cape of Storms, is notoriously treacherous for ships, and in 1657, a Dutch vessel was wrecked in what is today Table Bay. The crew of the vessel were the first to attempt to settle in the Cape.

Shortly thereafter, the Dutch East India Company was formed, and a permanent settlement was established in the area under the command of Jan Van Riebeeck. It became the main trading post on the spice route to India. From the beginning, the trade relationship with the indigenous KhoiKhoi was marked with conflict. The Dutch settlers expanded and began to establish farms, which encroached on the nomadic territories of the KhoiKhoi. The original Dutch settlers were joined by German and French Huguenots, who were mostly Calvinists fleeing persecution by King Louis XIV.

Jan van Riebeeck began to import slaves from Madagascar and Indonesia, and the growing population resulted in the inevitable expansion of land procurement and conflict with the KhoiKhoi. The settlers drove the indigenous people from their traditional land, decimated them with superior weapons, and introduced diseases. Most survivors became slaves, and over time, unions occurred between the black slaves and white owners, whose descendants are the colored race of South Africa today.

British Rule

By the end of the 18th century, the Dutch mercantile power began to fade and the British moved in to fill the gap. They seized the Cape in 1795, and British sovereignty was recognized in 1815 by the Congress of Vienna. The British established a colony at the Cape. White supremacy reigned, and differentiation based on race was deeply entrenched. Outside of the Cape

Colony, groups of white Dutch pastoralists and black communities populated the country. This effectively created two groups of white peoples: the Dutch, who were the ancestors of today's Afrikaans people, and the British, who were the forerunners of South Africa's English population.

The English-speaking British dominated the towns, politics, trade, finance, and mining, while the Dutch, who became known as the Burghers or Boers, remained farmers. These two groups lived in conflict as their religious and political ideals clashed. Although slavery was abolished in 1834, British conservatism did little to encourage racial reforms, and white dominance remained.

The Zulu Nation

The Zulu people today are native to the province of KwaZulu-Natal. They are historically a mighty warrior nation who populated the east coast of South Africa as early as the 16th century. Border disputes between the British and Dutch colonists and the African people characterized the early history. These disputes escalated in the 19th century, resulting in immense upheavals with great loss of life between both the British and the Dutch, whose ideologies conflicted, and the indigenous people. The Zulu nation, which up until the early 19th century existed as disparate kingdoms, organized themselves into a unified, centralized, and militaristic state under King Shaka Zulu.

The Afrikaner

At this time, the Dutch farmers, known as the Boers, were growing increasing dissatisfied with British supremacy, and several groups banded together and began what became known as the Great Trek, a journey from the coast northward into the interior in search of greater independence. Known as the pioneers or the *Voortrekkers,* they encountered little resistance from the indigenous plains peoples, with the exception of the Zulu nation in Zululand, Natal.

Zulu-Boer wars ensued with losses experienced on both sides, but the Boers finally succeeded in slaughtering the Zulus with superior arms at the Battle of Blood River.

The British, however, prevented the Boers from establishing an independent state in Natal, and the Boers were forced further inland into the arid central region of the Karoo of the Orange Free State. The Boers continued to increase their settlements and with the influx of Indian workers, resentment between the Boers and the British grew, resulting in a number of Anglo-Boer wars. These ended with a Boer victory in 1881 and the establishment of the South African Republic with Paul Kruger as president. With the discovery of South African mineral wealth, the British fought back, eventually defeating the Boers and by 1902, British sovereignty had been reestablished. The Boer nation, however, refused to be anglicized by the British and continued to establish pockets of independent nationalist groups with the Afrikaans language as the symbol of Afrikaner nationhood.

The British unionized all the colonies in 1909 under British rule, but with home rule for the Afrikaners. This system left the indigenous and black people completely marginalized. All indigenous people were denied access to parliament. The Native Lands Act was passed in 1913 as the first official segregation act and remained in place until 1990. Under the act, the black tribes were severely restricted in land ownership and movement. British segregationist legislation formed the foundation for the apartheid government, depriving the black, colored, and Indian people of the right to vote. This effectively entrenched residential, social, educational, financial, and political segregation. The British were eventually overthrown by the Afrikaner government in 1948, headed by General Louis Botha, which resulted in the formalization of the apartheid system and the South African National Party.

Under Apartheid

Apartheid, which literally means "separateness," was a system of legal racial segregation enforced by the national party in power in South Africa until 1990, by which white minority rule was ensured. The legislation classified South Africans into racial groups. Black people were forcibly removed from their lands and settled in demarcated areas known as the townships, outside of the cities and away from services and facilities. Under apartheid, marriages and sexual relations between people of different races were prohibited, racial classification was formalized, and the black people were stripped of their citizenship and restricted to designated tribal homelands. Where one could live and with whom one could socialize, relate to, or marry was determined by race. Those who transgressed these rules were prosecuted; people were incarcerated, tortured, and sentenced to death. Families were split apart as breadwinners were forced to migrate from their homelands to the cities to find work.

Most important to our work here, all cultural, spiritual, and indigenous religious practices were illegal, and this included the African healing practices. Black people were forced to convert to Christianity, and missionary churches were set up in most of the tribal homelands. Apartheid South Africa also meant that cultural identities and practices, including the African or traditional healing system, were rendered criminal acts and prosecuted. Thus African healers are still often reluctant to document and share their practices with Western people. There remain residual superstitions, misperceptions, and misunderstandings of this realm.

The release of Nelson Mandela in 1990 signaled the beginning of the transition toward a democracy. It is only as recently as 2004 that the Department of Health, South Africa, passed the Traditional Health Practitioners Act and recognized the Council for Traditional Healers. There are approximately 250,000 known healers in the country, and approximately 85 percent of the population, predominantly black people, consult with them.

Notes

1. *Mama* (mother) is both a term of endearment and respect. All female healers are addressed in this way. Male healers are addressed in the masculine as *Baba* (father).
2. This anecdote took place during the apartheid regime of the old South African government. At that time, it was rare for white people to visit the designated townships of the black people and to be associated with the African healers.
3. To embrace the realm of the African healer in the complex context of South Africa requires a deep confrontation with the multifaceted and nuanced realm of culture and race. It is a complexity that confronts me daily, and its full extent remains forever beyond my reach as a white South African. I am further aware of my Western-based training that informs a certain way of thinking and presents me with a number of paradoxes of conceptualization. In an attempt to navigate these challenges, I have drawn from my experiences of living and working within a culture that is not my birth culture. By definition, I remain the observer, and at times, the interloper.
4. During apartheid, the practices of the African healers were outlawed and vilified, deeply embedded in ignorance and prejudice of white colonial South Africa. Today this has changed somewhat. African healing practices are no longer illegal; nonetheless, residual misperceptions remain. In 2004, the Department of Health, South Africa, passed legislation—the Traditional Health Practitioners Act—and recognized the Council for Traditional Healers. However, there is still conflict between the church, biomedical realms, and indigenous systems, and white *sangomas* are still relatively unusual.
5. The initiation is a demanding and difficult process that unfolds over a number of years and requires the development of sufficient ego strength

in order to integrate and withstand the powerful constellation of unconscious archetypal energies without becoming identified with these forces, inflated, or suffering a defeat or psychotic break. Many do not succeed.

6. In direct translation, *Ntombi* means "young girl or daughter." My patient felt this was an appropriate pseudonym as it seemed symbolic of how she began the process: undifferentiated, unformed, without an identity.

7. Jung used the term God-image to refer to an image of the totality, in other words to refer to an image of the Self. Jung (1948a, para 528) explained the difference between his understanding of the concept of God, as a theological concept, and the God-image. Psychologically, the God-image suggests an inner experience of that which holds the highest value for the individual, and is not to be conflated with the concept of God as a religious idea, although for the individual to catch a glimpse of the Self is undoubtedly a numinous experience, which has a religious quality. Jung also showed how the contents of the collective unconscious influence the collective consciousness of the day and how the changing God-image is expressed in the historical development of each aeon.

8. All quotes, reflections, and explanations are from personal communications with various healers in the author's archives unless otherwise stated. All are senior healers or initiates who continue to actively engage in healing as well as in initiatory practices in various contexts, including rural and urban settings in South and southern Africa.

9. Jung's use of the term *primitive* requires comment. In 21st century cultural and socio-political awareness, the term *primitive* denotes extremely pejorative connotations of racism, prejudice, and ignorance. It is beyond the scope of this book to enter into a meaningful discussion of the implications of this, or even to claim to "know" what Jung meant with his use of the word. Suffice it to note here that in my experience, indigenous cultures seem to retain a nuanced and differentiated relationship with the deep strata of the autonomous psyche that is often lacking in Western cultures. One motivation in writing this book is my attempt to demonstrate this and to provide a small counterfoil to Jung's perhaps undifferentiated and limited experience in this regard, which was representative of the zeitgeist of his time.

10. This form of healing ceremony is found across most of the Nguni tribes. In the Xhosa tradition, it is known as the *xhentsa*, as documented by Vera Buhrmann in her book *Living between Two Worlds* (1984).

11. *Mutus Liber* or "Mute book" is a hermetic philosophical work published in 1677. It consists of 28 plates or illustrations without words and is subject to various interpretations. Its authorship is unclear but largely attributed to Altus Eli Luminusus Aequalis. Jung studied the *Mutus Liber* and he interpreted the images to depict the stages of the alchemical opus.

12. One aim of alchemy in relation to the *coniunctio*, according to Jung, is to beget the light in the shape of the *filius philosophorum*. Jung, in the chapter titled "The Components of the *Coniunctio*" in *Mysterium coniunctionis* (1955–56), explained: "Above all, the prima materia is the mother of the lapis, the *filius philosophorum*" (para. 14); and "the secret hidden in matter, the "light above all lights" (para. 34). For further discussion of this complex concept, the reader is directed to Jung's *Mysterium Coniunctionis*.

13. The transference and countertransference are often a central phenomenon in the analytical opus, and central, too, to the formation of the therapeutic vessel and as a phenomenon of transformation. Jung, in the foreword to "The Psychology of the Transference," noted in relation to the process of the transference that it "often presents a difficult problem . . . and that the success or failure of the treatment appears to be bound up with it in a very fundamental way" (1946b, pp. 164–65). Jung continued to explain the link between the phenomenon of the transference and the symbolism of alchemy, particularly with respect to the symbolism of the *coniunctio* often symbolized by the mystical marriage and contrasexual opposites, the anima and animus. The anima is the unconscious personality in men and finds expression mainly in specific moods, erotic fantasies, and emotional incentives for life. The animus in women appears as unconscious impulses to action, opinions, and convictions. These contrasexual aspects are often projected onto the other and form a bridge to relationships. These are fundamental concepts in Jung's psychology, but are not a focus of this work. For a full explanation of the anima and animus, and transference and countertransference in Jungian psychology, see Jung (1943; 1946b).

14. Jung notes that the phenomenon of dismemberment is integral to the alchemical process. In relation to the alchemical operation of the *solutio*, Jung (1955–56) explained that "water . . . has that decomposing and dissolving property which anticipates the . . . dismemberment" (para. 361). For a further description of the symbolism of dismemberment, see also Jung (1954c).

15. I have not come across a formal sacrificial ritual that embodies the number two or that specifically takes place over two days. The two suggests differentiation and a duality. As the overall intention of the initiation per se, of which these sacrificial ceremonies are a part, strives for a union of opposites, it is possible that a ritual symbolizing the two would not be relevant.

16. The spirit Mercurius is a vast and complex phenomenon that is central to both the alchemical opus and Jung's analytical psychology. Essentially, Jung identified the mercurial essence as the "*principium individuationis*," the principle of individuation (1948g, para. 244). The spirit Mercurius embodies opposites as both the *prima materia* and the ultimate outcome of the opus: spirit and matter, dark and light; Sol and Luna—a paradoxical and autonomous spirit of nature, or psychologically, the objective psyche. For a more extensive explanation, see Jung (1948g).

17. The reader is directed to Jung's autobiography *Memories, Dreams and Reflections* as well as *The Red Book* for a more in-depth exploration of these figures as part of Jung's active imagination during the period wherein he formulated his concepts of the archetypes of the collective unconscious.

18. The multicolored apparel of the healer is not characteristically always found in the Zulu tradition, where the focus is predominantly on the red and white. Examples of the addition of many colors is more likely to be found in other traditions such as the Pondo clan of the Eastern Cape, South Africa. However, for Ntombi, her dreams seemed to demand this additional feature.

19. The reader is directed to Marie-Louise von Franz' works *Number and Time* (1974) as well as *Psyche and Matter* (1992) for further discussion of these principles.

20. The reader is directed to Jung's work on alchemy in the *Collected Works*, volumes 12, 13, and 14 for in-depth discussion on the symbolism of the *coniunctio*, which is beyond the scope of this book. From a psychological understanding, the *coniunctio* also symbolizes the union of opposites of the anima/animus (the contrasexual psychic aspects of the masculine and feminine respectively) and is often represented by numerous motifs of the *hieros gamos*, the mystical marriage, the bride and bridegroom, Sol and Luna, and spirit and matter, among others.

References

American Psychiatric Association. (2013). *Diagnostic and Statistical Manual of Mental Disorders,* Fifth Edition. Arlington, VA: American Psychiatric Association

Apt, T. (2005). *Introduction to picture interpretation according to C.G. Jung.* Zurich, Switzerland: Living Human Heritage Publications.

Bohm, D. (1980). *Wholeness and implicate order.* London, UK: Kegan Paul.

Buhrmann, V. (1984). *Living between Two Worlds.* Cape Town, South Africa: Human and Rousseau.

Campbell, J. (1968). *Hero with a thousand faces.* NJ: Princeton University Press.

Corbin, H. (1964). Mundus imaginalis or the imaginary and the imaginal. *Cahiers Internationaux de Symbolisme 6*, 3–26.

de Vries, A. (1974). *Dictionary of symbols and imagery.* Amsterdam, The Netherlands: North-Holland.

Edinger, E. (1972). *Ego and archetype.* Boston, MA: Shambhala.

Edinger, E. (1984). *Creation of consciousness: Jung's myth for modern man.* Toronto, Canada: Inner City Books.

Edinger, E. (1991). *Anatomy of the psyche: Alchemical symbolism in psychotherapy.* LaSalle, IL: Open Court.

Edinger, E. (1995). *The mysterium lectures: A journey through C.G. Jung's "Mysterium coniunctionis."* Toronto, Canada: Inner City Books.

Edinger, E. (1996). *The new God-image.* Wilmette, IL: Chiron Publications.

Eliade, M. (1958). *Patterns in comparative religion.* NJ: Princeton University Press.

Eliade, M. (1972). *Archaic techniques of ecstasy.* NJ: Princeton University Press.

Eliade, M. (1989). *Shamanism: Archaic techniques of ecstasy.* London, UK: Arkana.

Hannah, B. (1981). *Encounters with the soul: Active imagination as developed by C.G. Jung.* Boston, MA: Sigo Press.

Hannah, B. (2006). *The archetypal symbolism of animals.* Wilmette, IL: Chiron Publications.

Henderson, J., & Oakes, M. (1963). *The wisdom of the serpent: The myths of death, rebirth and resurrection.* New York, NY: Ambassador Books.

Jaffe, L. (1991). Transforming the God-image: An interview with Edward Edinger. *Psychological Perspectives, 25,* 40–51.

Jung, C.G. (1923/1971). *Psychological types. CW,* vol. 6. NJ: Princeton University Press.

Jung, C.G. (1931/1964). Mind and earth. In *CW,* vol. 10, *Civilization in transition.* NJ: Princeton University Press.

Jung, C.G. (1934a/1969). Basic postulates of analytical psychology. In *CW,* vol. 8, *The Structure and Dynamics of the Psyche.* NJ: Princeton University Press.

Jung, C.G. (1934b/1964). The meaning of psychology for modern man. In *CW,* vol. 10, *Civilization in transition.* NJ: Princeton University Press.

Jung, C.G. (1937/1954). The realities of practical psychotherapy. In *CW,* vol. 16, *The practice of psychotherapy.* NJ: Princeton University Press.

Jung, C.G. (1938/1968). Psychological aspects of the mother archetype. In *CW,* vol. 9i, *Archetypes and the collective unconscious.* NJ: Princeton University Press.

Jung, C.G. (1939/1976). The symbolic life. In *CW,* vol. 18, *The Symbolic Life.* NJ: Princeton University Press.

Jung, C.G. (1940/1969). Psychology and religion. In *CW,* vol. 11, *Psychology and Religion.* NJ: Princeton University Press.

Jung, C.G. (1942/1967). Paracelsus as a spiritual phenomenon. In *CW,* vol. 13, *Alchemical studies.* Princeton, NJ: Princeton University Press.

Jung, C.G. (1943). On the psychology of the unconscious, In *CW,* vol. 7, Two essays on analytical psychology.

Jung, C.G. (1944/1968). *Psychology and alchemy. CW,* vol. 12. NJ: Princeton University Press.

June, C.G. (1946a/1964). The undiscovered self. In *CW,* vol. 10, *Civilization in transition.* NJ: Princeton University Press.

Jung, C.G. (1946b/1954). The psychology of the transference. In *CW,* vol. 16, *The practice of psychotherapy.* NJ: Princeton University Press.

Jung, C.G. (1946c/1954). Psychotherapy and a philosophy of life. In *CW*, vol. 16, *The practice of psychotherapy*. NJ: Princeton University Press.

Jung, C.G. (1948a/1969). On psychic energy. In *CW*, vol. 8, *The Structure and Dynamics of the Psyche*. NJ: Princeton University Press.

Jung, C.G. (1948b/1969). On the nature of dreams. In *CW*, vol. 8, *The Structure and Dynamics of the Psyche*. NJ: Princeton University Press.

Jung, C.G. (1948c/1969). A psychological approach to the dogma of the Trinity. In *CW*, vol. 11, *Psychology and Religion*. NJ: Princeton University Press.

Jung, C.G. (1948d/1969). The psychological foundations of belief in spirits. In *CW*, vol. 8, *The Structure and Dynamics of the Psyche*. NJ: Princeton University Press.

Jung, C.G. (1948e/1976). Psychology and spiritualism. In *CW*, vol. 18, *The Symbolic Life*. NJ: Princeton University Press.

Jung, C.G. (1948f). Short report of Prof. Jung's remarks after Mrs. Carol F. Baumann's lecture on "Some implications of extra sensory perception." Report of the Rhine Experiments at Duke University, June 5, 1948. Unpublished material.

Jung, C.G. (1948g/1967). The spirit Mercurius. In *CW*, vol. 13, *Alchemical studies*. NJ: Princeton University Press.

Jung, C.G. (1951/1959). *Aion*. *CW*, vol. 9ii. NJ: Princeton University Press.

Jung, C.G. (1952a/1969). Answer to Job. In *CW*, vol. 11, *Psychology and Religion*. NJ: Princeton University Press.

Jung, C.G. (1952b/1956). *Symbols of transformation*. *CW*, vol. 5. NJ: Princeton University Press.

Jung, C.G. (1952c/1969). Synchronicity: An acausal connecting principle. In *CW*, vol. 8, *The Structure and Dynamics of the Psyche*. NJ: Princeton University Press.

Jung, C.G. (1953/1969). Psychological commentary on *The Tibetan Book of the Dead*. In *CW*, vol. 11, *Psychology and Religion*. NJ: Princeton University Press.

Jung, C.G. (1954a/1969). On the nature of the psyche. In *CW*, vol. 8, *The Structure and Dynamics of the Psyche*. NJ: Princeton University Press.

Jung, C.G. (1954b/1967). The philosophical tree. In *CW*, vol. 13, *Alchemical studies*. NJ: Princeton University Press.

Jung, C.G. (1954c/1969). Transformation symbolism in the mass. In *CW*, vol. 11, *Psychology and Religion*. NJ: Princeton University Press.

Jung, C.G. (1954d/1969). A psychological approach to the trinity. In *CW*, vol. 11, *Psychology and Religion*. NJ: Princeton University Press.

Jung, C.G. (1954e/1967). The visions of Zosimos. In *CW*, vol. 13, *Alchemical studies*. NJ: Princeton University Press.

Jung, C.G. (1955/1968). Mandalas. In *CW*, vol. 9i, *Archetypes and the collective unconscious*. NJ: Princeton University Press.

Jung, C.G. (1955–56/1970). *Mysterium coniunctionis*. *CW*, vol. 14. NJ: Princeton University Press.

Jung, C.G. (1957a/1967). Commentary on "The Secret of the Golden Flower." In *CW*, vol. 13, *Alchemical studies*. NJ: Princeton University Press.

Jung, C.G. (1957b/1964). The undiscovered self (present and future). In *CW*, vol. 10, *Civilization in transition*. NJ: Princeton University Press.

Jung, C.G. (1958/1969). The transcendent function. In *CW*, vol. 8, *The Structure and Dynamics of the Psyche*. NJ: Princeton University Press.

Jung, C.G. (1958b/1964). Flying saucers: A modern myth. In *CW*, vol. 10, *Civilization in transition*. NJ: Princeton University Press.

Jung, C.G. (1961a). *Memories, dreams, reflections*. New York, NY: Random House.

Jung, C.G. (1961b/1976). Symbols and the interpretation of dreams. In *CW*, vol. 18, *The Symbolic Life*. NJ: Princeton University Press.

Jung, C.G. (1962). *The secret of the golden flower*. London, UK: Routledge and Kegan Paul.

Jung, C.G. (1966). The structure of the unconscious. In *CW* , vol. 7, *Two Essays on Analytical Psychology*. NJ: Princeton University Press.

Jung, C.G. (1973). *Letters, 1906–1950* (R.F.C. Hull, trans.). NJ: Princeton University Press.

Jung, C.G. (1975). *Letters, 1951–1961* (R.F.C. Hull, trans.). NJ: Princeton University Press.

Jung, C.G. (1977). *C.G. Jung speaking: Interviews and encounters*. NJ: Princeton University Press.

Jung, C.G. (1989). *Introduction to Jungian psychology: Notes of the seminar on analytical psychology given in 1925*. NJ: Princeton University Press.

Jung, C.G. (1990). *Man and his symbols*. London, UK: Arkana Books.

Jung, C.G. (1997a). *Vision seminars* (Vol. 1). NJ: Princeton University Press.
Jung, C.G. (1997b). *Vision seminars* (Vol. 2). NJ: Princeton University Press.

Jung, C.G. (2008). *Children's dreams* (L. Jung & M. Meyer-Grass, Eds.; E. Falzeder & T. Woolfson, Trans.). NJ: Princeton University Press.

Jung, C.G. (2009). *The red book: Liber Novus*. Sonu Shamdasani (Ed.). New York: Philemon Press.

Meier, C.A. (1984). *Ancient incubation and modern psychology.* (David Roscoe, trans.). Einsiedeln, Switzerland: Diamon Press.

Meier, C.A. (1989). *Healing dream ritual: Ancient incubation and modern psychotherapy.* Einsiedeln, Switzerland: Daimon Press.

Mutwa, C. (1996). *The song of the stars.* New York, NY: Barrytown Press.

Neumann, E. (1954). *The origins and history of consciousness.* NJ: Princeton University Press.

Neumann, E. (1955). *The great mother*. NJ: Princeton University Press.

Otto, R. (1958). The idea of the holy. London: Oxford University Press.

Peek, P. (1991). *African divination systems: Ways of knowing*. Bloomington: Indiana University Press.

Radomsky, L. (2006). Global health crisis: Can indigenous healing practices offer a valuable resource? *International Journal of Disability, Development and Education.* 53(4). p. 212.

Radomsky, L. (2009). White skin, black soul: Initiation and integration in African traditional healing. *Jung Journal: Culture and Psyche, 3*(3), 33–43.

Radomsky, L., & Levers, L. L. (2012). Voices of the African traditional healer: Implications for cross cultural educational practices. In A. S. Yeung, C.F.K. Lee, & E. L. Brown (Eds.), *International advances in education: Global initiatives for equity and social Justice* (Vol. 7, pp. 79–100). Charlotte, NC: Information Age Publishing.

Radomsky, L. (2017). African healing, sacrifice, number symbolism, and the psychology of C.G. Jung. *Psychological Perspectives.* 60(1), 53–67.

Ronnberg, A. (ed.). (2010). *The book of symbols: Reflections on archetypal images.* Cologne, Germany: Taschen.

Rossi, E. L. (2008). Conversations with Marie-Louise von Franz at 70. *Psychological Perspectives, 17*(2), 151–160.

Samuels, A., Shorter, B., & Plaut, F. (1991). *A critical dictionary of Jungian analysis.* London, UK: Routledge.

von Franz, M.-L. (1970). *The interpretation of fairy tales*. Dallas, TX: Spring Publications.

von Franz, M.-L. (1974). *Number and time* (A. Dykes, Trans.). Evanston, IL: Northwestern University Press.

von Franz, M.-L. (1980a). *Alchemy: An introduction to the symbolism and the psychology*. Toronto, Canada: Inner City Books.

von Franz, M.-L. (1980b). *On divination and synchronicity: The psychology of meaning and chance.* Toronto, Canada: Inner City Books.

von Franz, M.-L. (1982). *The feminine in fairy tales*. Boston, MA: Shambhala.

von Franz, M.-L. (1987). *On dreams and death* (E. X. Kennedy & V. Brooks, Trans.). Boston, MA: Shambhala.

von Franz, M.-L. (1992). *Psyche and matter.* Boston, MA: Shambhala.

von Franz, M.-L. (1997a). *Archetypal dimensions of the psyche*. Boston, MA: Shambhala.

von Franz, M.-L. (1997b). *Archetypal patterns in fairy tales*. Toronto, Canada: Inner City Books.

von Franz, M.-L. (1997c). *Alchemical active imagination*. Boston, MA: Shambhala.

Von Franz, M.-L. (1998). *C.G. Jung: His myth in our time* (W. Kennedy, Trans.). Toronto, Canada: Inner City Books.

von Franz, M.-L. (1999). *The cat: A tale of feminine redemption*. Toronto, Canada: Inner City Books.

von Franz, M.-L. (2008). Consciousness, power and sacrifice. *Psychological Perspectives 8*(2), 378.

Whitney, M. (Director). (1986). *Matter of heart* (DVD). C.G. Jung Institute of Los Angeles.

Wosien, M.-G. (1974). *Sacred dance: Encounter with the gods*. London, UK: Thames and Hudson.

Index